Integrating Social Support in Nursing

MIRIAM J. STEWART

(1993).

SAGE Publications
International Educational and Professional Publisher
Newbury Park London New Delhi

For information address:

SAGE Publications, Inc.
2455 Teller Road
Newbury Park, California 91320

SAGE Publications Ltd.
6 Bonhill Street
London EC2A 4PU
United Kingdom

SAGE Publications India Pvt. Ltd.
M-32 Market
Greater Kailash I
New Delhi 110 048 India

Printed in the United States of America

Library of Congress Cataloging-in-Publication Data

Stewart, Miriam (Miriam Joyce)
Integrating social support in nursing / Miriam J. Stewart.
p. cm.
Includes bibliographical references and index.
ISBN 0-8039-4273-7 (cl). — ISBN 0-8039-4274-5 (pb)
1. Patients—Social networks. 2. Nursing—Psychological aspects.
3. Nursing—Philosophy. I. Title.
RA418.S824 1993
610.73′01—dc20 93-1201

93 94 95 96 97 10 9 8 7 6 5 4 3 2 1

Sage Production Editor: Diane S. Foster

Contents

Acknowledgments

It is gratifying to acknowledge the sage advice of Dr. Benjamin Gottlieb, Dr. Jane Norbeck, and Dr. Virginia Tilden, who guided and supported my interest in the significance of social support for nursing. Benjamin Gottlieb, Ph.D. (Professor in the Department of Psychology, University of Guelph, and Director of the Gerontology Research Centre), an internationally renowned scholar, has published 3 books and more than 50 papers on social support and has received extensive funding for his research. Jane S. Norbeck, R.N., D.N.Sc., F.A.A.N. (Professor and Dean, School of Nursing, University of California, San Francisco), a renowned contributor to the nursing literature on social support, developed a major social support measure and initiated the two international nursing conferences on social support research. Virginia Tilden, D.N.Sc., R.N., F.A.A.N. (Professor and Associate Dean for Research, School of Nursing; Program Director for Family Health Research Training, Oregon Health Sciences University), created a social support instrument that has been tested and used internationally and contributed to the conceptualization of the construct. I record grateful recognition of Roberta Emms's and Paulette Skerrett's skill and perseverance in typing this book. Finally, I wish to thank Sharon Alexander, M.A. (Psychology), whose tireless efforts and creative energy yielded the extensive background research and references for several chapters. This book is dedicated to my daughters, Evelyn and Shauna, and to my parents, Ross and Dorothy Mortimer—my significant sources of support.

Foreword

During the past 20 years the concept of social support has been front and center for a great number of social and health scientists. Its allure stems in part from the clear evidence that the personal community in which people are enveloped has a profound impact on their health and morale, and in part from the recognition that practical steps can be taken to mobilize and augment support on behalf of populations at risk. In addition, social support has captured the attention of policy makers in the health and social services fields because mutual aid and informal care are indispensable complements to the programs provided by local and federal governments. Without the help and emotional aid rendered by the community's informal support systems, institutional resources would be overwhelmed, and indicators of health and well-being would decline precipitously.

This volume traces the particular significance of social support for researchers and practitioners in the field of nursing. It spotlights the contributions nurses have made to our understanding and measurement of social support, and it points the way toward new initiatives nurses can take to augment and fortify the support that people gain from their social networks and from the settings in which nurses practice. Equally important, the volume firmly embeds social support in nursing theory and, in doing so, enriches the pedagogy and training of nurses, while enlarging the conceptual framework that guides their practice.

Dr. Miriam Stewart is superbly qualified to author this definitive treatise. As the architect of the Social Support Research Program at Dalhousie University's School of Nursing, she has been responsible for launching a wide-ranging series of investigations touching on stress, social support, and coping. This work has given her a commanding view of the challenges attending the investigation and modification of social support. Moreover, her breadth of vision and the unbridled enthusiasm she brings to her leadership have ensured that this research program embraces a large, interdisciplinary group of scientists and practitioners.

Researchers will find this volume thick in research and cogent in its interpretation. Dr. Stewart presents a careful appraisal of the existing literature, showing commendable skill in unraveling a tangled skein of empirical evidence. Moreover, her vigorous efforts to bring diverse theoretical viewpoints to bear on the various facets of social support are especially impressive and laudable. Brushing the earth from the rock, Dr. Stewart also lays bare a set of intervention strategies that can be applied in diverse health contexts and among contrasting patient and community populations. She is particularly insightful about how the process of marshalling social support differs in the context of acute versus chronic illness. Above all, she conveys a strong and clear message about the importance of structuring interventions so nurses become partners rather than providers in the enterprise of health care.

This book is much more than a chronicle of social support's application to the field of nursing. It is, in addition, a carefully thought out and persuasively argued set of ideas about the challenges that await nurses who wish to base their actions on a sound theoretical footing and who strive to place nursing practice in the vanguard of health care and health education. One cannot help but come away with a sense of urgency and excitement about the work that remains to be done to more fully explore the potential of social support for the field of nursing.

Benjamin H. Gottlieb
University of Guelph

❖ CHAPTER ONE ❖

Concepts and Controversies in Social Support

Introduction

> A newly divorced woman with a teenage child and a preschooler recently moved into a new neighborhood. Shortly after the move, Mary lost her job as a grocery store clerk and is struggling financially. Sean, her 4-year-old son, has developed problems with stuttering and her 13-year-old daughter, Shelley, is unhappy with her new school and misses her old friends. Mary's widowed mother lives across town. The children rarely see their father because of their mother's feelings of bitterness and betrayal. Social support has been demonstrated to enable people like Mary to cope with transitions and situational and maturational stressors. Yet support is complex and multifaceted, in part because members of Mary's social network, including children, mother, ex-husband, friends, and former work colleagues, may not necessarily be sources of support. Furthermore, the type of support provided may not be appropriate for the stress she is experiencing.

Social support has been the focus of commentary from varied disciplines over the past decade. In conventional terms, social support is assistance rendered by laypersons who are part of one's social network, rather than by professionals. More specifically, it is emotional, instrumental, informational, and appraisal assistance (House

& Kahn, 1985) provided by family, friends, neighbors, coworkers (Tardy, 1985), community leaders, indigenous lay helpers, volunteers, and self-help mutual-aid groups (Pearlin, 1985; Wills, 1985). In contrast, the assistance that professionals provide is best thought of as surrogate support, extending the support available in the client's network and replacing that which is not available (Norbeck, 1988b).

Social networks influence how their members seek help from professionals and use professional services by buffering experiences of stress, thereby eliminating the need for help; by providing support and services; by acting as screening and referral agents; and by transmitting values, attitudes, and norms about help seeking (Birkel & Repucci, 1983; Gourash, 1978). Lay networks also enhance, complement, or serve as alternatives to professional services (Whittaker & Garbarino, 1983).

Social support is a significant concept for nurses and other health professionals, because it influences not only health services use but also health behavior and health status. Although a comprehensive theory of social support has not yet been developed, operationalization of the construct and hypotheses regarding its impact on health have been proposed.

Diverse Definitions of the Construct

Social support can be interpreted from distinct yet interlocking theories generated by sociologists and psychologists. The burgeoning multidisciplinary focus on social support indicates a need to examine these differing perspectives and to extract pertinent commonalities and distinctions. Indeed, analysis and testing of the conceptual and theoretical underpinnings of social support proliferate in the nursing and social-psychological literatures. In particular, the conceptual distinctions between social support (as informal help) and formal services generate queries regarding requisite professional roles and relationships with lay networks.

Definitions are critical to descriptions of concepts. Unfortunately, many definitions of social support—some lacking explication and conceptual clarity, some somewhat circular—have been presented in the literature (see Table 1.1 for examples), illustrating the disparate views about the properties of this important concept. Gottlieb (1983) defines social support as "verbal and/or non-verbal information or advice, tangible aid, or action that is proffered by social intimates or inferred by their presence and has beneficial emotional or behavioral effects on the recipient" (pp. 28-29), thus usefully identifying type, source, and outcome of support. Shumaker and Brownell's (1984) definition of social support as "the exchange of resources between at least two individuals [that is] perceived by the provider or the recipient to be intended to enhance the well being of the recipient" (p. 13) explicates the critical bidirectional nature of social support implied by other authors. Pioneer authors in the social support field (e.g., Cassel, Cobb, and Caplan) all emphasized that some of the beneficial effects of social relationships are due to their buffering properties in the presence of stress (House, Landis, & Umberson, 1988).

These properties are elaborated and exemplified in prevalent typologies. Wortman (1984), drawing upon the taxonomies of authors of seminal works (Caplan, 1974; Cobb, 1976; House, 1981; Kahn & Antonucci, 1980; Kaplan, Cassel, & Gore, 1977; Weiss, 1974), identifies six types of social support: expression of positive affect, expression of agreement, encouragement of open expression of feelings, offer of advice and information, provision of material aid, and provision of information that the individual is part of a network of reciprocal help and mutual obligation. However, it could be legitimately argued that House (1981) subsumes significant subcomponents of diverse definitions in his all-encompassing categories of emotional, informational, instrumental, and appraisal support resources. Cutrona's (1990) review confirms five distinct dimensions of support: emotional, esteem (appraisal), tangible (instrumental), information, and social integration. This review adds the notion of integration within a network, thus combining structural (network) with functional (types of resources) characteristics of support.

Social support frequently is considered a multidimensional construct. The concept has been operationalized in divergent ways: quantity of connections, quality, utilization, meaning, availability, and satisfaction with support (Brownell & Shumaker, 1984; Sullivan & Poertner, 1989; Thoits, 1982). According to Antonucci (1985), the distinction between quality and quantity is well recognized, the former having greater impact on outcomes. Many have focused on perceived or subjective social support in cognitive terms; others emphasize the interpersonal transactions that reduce stress and enhance coping (e.g., Gottlieb, 1981; Wilcox & Vernberg, 1985). Most concur that social support refers to social transactions that are "perceived by

(text continued on page 6)

Table 1.1 Selected Definitions of Social Support (in chronological order)

Author	*Definition*	*Perspective/ Contributions*	*Limitations*
Caplan (1974)	"The primary group in which people participate affords them three kinds of support provisions: (a) the significant others help the individual mobilize his psychological resources and master his emotional burdens; (b) they share his tasks; and (c) they provide him with extra supplies of money, material tools, skills, and cognitive guidance to improve his handling of his situation" (p. 20).	Social psychiatry; social interaction; preventive and protection against disease	View of social support as commodity to be mobil-ized in crisis
Cobb (1976)	"Social support is conceived to be information belonging to one or more of the following three classes: (1) information leading the subject to believe he is cared for and loved; (2) information leading the subject to believe that he is esteemed and valued; (3) information leading the subject to believe that he belongs to a network of communication and mutual obligation" (p. 302).	Clinical medicine; cogni-tive perceptual; protective function of social support against pathological states; buffering effect; major role in coping process by con-trolling affect	Omitted tangible and limited support social support to intangible information
Kahn & Antonucci (1980); Antonucci (1985)	"Interpersonal transactions that include one or more of the following: The expression of positive affect of one person toward another, the affirmation or endorsement of another person's behavior, perceptions or expressed views; giving of symbolic or material aids to one another" (p.173) ."Convoy" or personal network changes throughout life span	Describe social support changes over time and life course; based on role and attachment theories	Superficial treatment of functions
Schaefer, Coyne, & Lazarus (1982)	Social support constitutes motional, informational, and tangible support: "an evaluation or appraisal of whether and to what extent an interaction or relationship is helpful."	Social interactions; concise, distinct subconcepts	Shallow

MacElveen-Hoehn & Eyers (1984)	"Information and resources from others in the environment that . . . minimize the perception of threat, maximize actual and perceived mastery, and facilitate direct action or anticipatory modes of coping" (p. 3).	Control and mastery	
Cohen & Syme (1985)	Resources provided by other persons	Concise, general; allows for possibility of negative as well as positive effects	Lacks explication of source, function, effect
Heller, Swindle, & Dusenbury (1986)	"A social activity is said to involve social support if it is perceived by the recipient of that activity as esteem enhancing or if it involved the provision of stress-related interpersonal aid (emotional support, cognitive restructuring, or instrumental aid)" (p. 467).	Elucidates impact of social support; acknowledges social activities	
Albrecht & Adelman (1987)	Verbal and nonverbal communication between recipients and providers that reduces uncertainty about the situation, the self, the other, or the relationship and functions to enhance a perception of personal control in one's life experience.	Control and mastery; communication; transactional process; dynamic interaction and mutual influence	
Gottlieb & Selby (1989)	Social support refers to processes of interaction in relationships and social structures that shore up coping, esteem, belonging, and competence through actual or predictable exchanges of tangible or psychosocial resources.	Emphasizes bidirectional exchange; acknowledges anticipated and actual social support; social support expressed in relationships	
Dunkel-Schetter & Skokan (1990)	Dyadic interactions in which one person attempts to provide information, assistance, or emotional support.	Focus on social interactions	Limited to two-person relationships; ignores appraisal support and reciprocity
Vaux (1990)	A meta construct with three distinct conceptual components: support network resources, supportive behavior, and subjective appraisals of support.	Comprehensive linking of objective and subjective components	Lacks specificity regarding resources and sources

the recipient or intended by the provider to facilitate coping in everyday life, and especially in response to stressful situations" (Pierce, Sarason, & Sarason, 1990). Other commonalities within definitions include the assumptions that social support refers to interpersonal interactions that provide emotional support or actual tangible help or information from members of the individual's social network, and that it is both given and received by the members of the network, creating a sense of belonging or social integration (Dimond, 1985; Norbeck & Tilden, 1988).

Nevertheless, absence of theoretical grounding is common and weakens definitions (Stewart, 1989b; Tilden, 1985c). Some argue that a global concept of social support should be replaced by precise concepts and models (Barrera, 1986; Coyne & Bulger, 1990; Dunkel-Schetter & Bennett, 1990; Heller, Swindle, & Dusenbury, 1986). Thus, the cognitive (perceived) and behavioral (received) constructs should be distinguished.

Heller et al. (1986) purport that we need better theoretical descriptions of the basic operating mechanisms of social support and of its component processes. Two common hypotheses are proposed by Newcomb (1990): "social support should be moderately stable across time and developmental periods; social support changes as a result of transactions between a person and the social environment" (p. 479). Rarely do definitions encompass determinants or outcomes of support (Tilden, 1985c). A broader theory of social support must address the quantity of social relationships, their formal structure, the content of these relationships (House, Landis, & Umberson, 1988), and a better understanding of the processes linked to health (Sarason, Sarason, & Pierce, 1990). Pierce et al. (1990) contend that social support is a product of interacting influences among persons, their personal relationships, and relevant situations. Some approaches emphasize the transaction and the dynamics of giving and receiving support in relationships (e.g., Gottlieb, 1988a; Gottlieb & Wagner, 1991; Heller, 1990; Hobfoll & Stokes, 1988). Most definitions have included functional effects for recipients and providers (primarily the former) and have been predominantly positive (Albrecht & Adelman, 1987). According to Vaux (1990), "The support process does not occur in a vacuum. Rather it takes place within a social ecology and is shaped by characteristics of the person . . . and the social context" (p. 510).

Social support for the purposes of this book is defined as

> interactions with family members, friends, peers, and health care providers that communicate information, esteem, aid, and reliable alliance. These communications improve coping, moderate the impact of stressors, and promote health. Social support occurs as a by-product of people's ongoing interactions. However, we cannot assume that it is accessible or beneficial. Instead, it is important to understand how supportive interactions are elicited with different associates, forms of expression of social support, and how social support can be miscarried or dissipate over time.

Researchers have studied the social support construct primarily from three perspectives: network structure, support functions, and the nature of relationships. Sociologists and anthropologists are intrigued by the structure of the basic ties between members of the social network. Like epidemiologists, they also have examined the functions of supportive resources (House, 1981; Weiss, 1974) that flow through these network ties. Psychologists have tended to emphasize *micro-level* analysis of the degree of attachment and nature of the focal individual's contact with network members in dyadic intimate relationships (Gottlieb, 1983, 1985a). One form of reciprocal relationship is the intimate (communal) relationship, in which members are concerned about each other's needs, rather than explicit exchanges (Clark, 1983). Intimacy involves investment, interactions, interdependence, self-disclosure, and warmth or affection (Perlman & Fehr, 1987).

In addition to the micro level of intimate relationships, Gottlieb (1983, 1985b) refers to the *mezzo level:* the prosocial resources, structure, and function of the social network of primary-group members, such as family. The altruistic, as distinct from the intimate, relationship (Hatfield & Sprecher, 1983) is typified by prosocial behavior, acts that benefit others than the actor (Baron & Byrne, 1977). Support provision is generally motivated by altruistic intentions (Dunkel-Schetter & Skokan, 1990). Four categories of prosocial behavior are comforting, cooperating, helping, and sharing (Burleson, 1982). The development of empathy, a significant component of prosocial and altruistic behavior, increases with advancing maturity and potentiates later access to social support (Gottlieb, 1983; Hatfield & Sprecher, 1983). Support is frequently conceived as an empathic communication process (Albrecht & Adelman, 1987). Shumaker and Brownell (1984) and Rook (1985) claim that research on prosocial behavior has implications for social support in terms of the helper's need to feel important to others; the impact of mood, values, and setting on the provider's decision to proffer assistance; and the possibility of diffusion of responsibility in large, dense networks.

Social-integration and community-participation links are measured at the macro level. Thus, network analysts have used a social-ecological approach rather than a personal-attributes approach in studying social support.

Distinctions Between Social Network and Social Support

Network size has been associated with amount of support (Hall & Wellman, 1985) and positive outcomes (Wortman, 1984). However, social network and social support are different concepts, as social networks may be sources of both stress and support (Berkman, 1985; Gottlieb, 1983; Wellman, 1981). Unfortunately, social networks and social support are sometimes confounded in the social-support literature and should be distinguished.

Social networks can serve functions of support yet can inhibit as well as facilitate supportive behaviors and relationships (Kaplan, Cassel, & Gore, 1977). They may not be voluntaristic (Wellman, 1982). These complex linkages can be expressive and horizontal to family and friends, or instrumental and vertical to the larger community and society (Wellman, 1985). This may be a false dichotomy, however, as family and friends frequently provide tangible support; and the appropriateness of horizontal and vertical ties are less clear than Kahn and Antonucci's (1980) notion of a "convoy" or concentric circles around persons, which represent decreasing levels of intimacy and contact in relationships.

Cohen and Syme (1985) distinguish the structure of an interpersonal relationship or network from the functions served by the relationship or network. Network analysts define the social network alternatively as the infrastructure of support, a set of nodes tied by specific types of relations, or the structure existing among a set of relations (Albrecht & Adelman, 1987; Hall & Wellman, 1985; House & Kahn, 1985). The network approach attends to the social matrix of supportive efforts and is based on the assumption that quantitative aspects of the social environment influence interactions among network members (Gottlieb, 1981; Pierce et al., 1990). It emphasizes the interpersonal context of support. Communication channels in networks are examined (Hall & Wellman, 1985), because they enable acquisition of social skills and reduce uncertainty. One complex conceptualization is that networks are the macro-level manifestation over time of dyadic interactions that embed the individual (Albrecht & Adelman, 1987). Four types of networks are identified by Bernard et al. (1990): the emotional support group composed of a few intimates, the larger social support group involving reciprocity of favors, the global network encompassing the first two and consisting of all people known to an individual, and the network of those outside the global network who could provide information about community resources. This typology reflects the convoy.

Structure of Networks

Structure includes social integration and social networks. Structure has effects through social regulation or control, relational demands and conflicts, and social support. The last, according to House, Umberson, & Landis (1988), pertains only to the "emotionally or instrumentally sustaining quality of social relationships." This distinction between support and network is useful. Social structure variables that influence support are size of community, socioeconomic status, ethnicity, age, marital status, and gender (House Umberson, & Landis, 1988). For example, women have greater sensitivity to needs of themselves and others, capacity to provide support, and dependence on support for psychological well-being (Flaherty & Richman, 1989).

Sources of support emerge from social networks. The source dimension of measurement instruments is one crude indicator of the presence or absence of a network and its size. House and Kahn (1985) recommend that the subject name only five persons closest to them. Others distinguish between support from key sources and support from all sources. Both strategies are considered valid by Norbeck (1985b) and Tardy (1985). In fact, a combined approach might provide the most relevant responses.

Tardy (1985) suggested that family, close friends, neighbors, coworkers, community, and professionals are members of support networks. The differentiation of friends from confidants or close friends seems useful. Griffith (1985) found that friends and spouses account for the largest proportion of social support providers; sources of support cited less often were (in order) other relatives, church members, coworkers, and professional caregivers. Thus, the distinction made earlier in this chapter that health professionals and other professionals are a legitimate source of temporary surrogate support, which should be considered along with or secondary to the more usual lay sources of social support, seems to hold true. In sum, a network perspective can delineate social worlds of individuals and a broad range of social processes.

Functions of Support

The functional content of relationships involves flows of types of resources. These resources are elaborated in different typologies (e.g., practical, emotional, informational, and appraisal) of support, as noted earlier. Assessment of kinds of support being provided helps to identify the clinical possibilities for intervention (Cohen & Syme, 1985; House & Kahn, 1985). The specific resource provided may or may not beneficially affect well-being depending on its appropriateness for the person and situation. For example, the information involved in appraisal support is relevant to self-evaluation and social comparison.

The functional approach thus focuses on social functions of network members and suggests that needs for support functions vary with stressors. It examines the role of situational factors in determining the nature and impact of transactions. As Dimond and Jones (1983) noted in their theoretical review, "The kind of support appropriate for a given situation is influenced at least in part by the nature of the stressful situation, the timing of support and the resources of the affected person" (p. 241). However, this approach of necessity fails to consider the sources of social support or the interpersonal context of social provisions (Pierce et al., 1990). Emergent debate, relevant to the functional approach, focuses on whether support is a unidimensional (e.g., Brown, 1986b) or multidimensional construct (e.g., Barrera, 1986).

Distinct Dimensions of Social Support

Cohen and Syme (1985) convincingly contend that six questions constitute the major conceptual issues in the study of social support: "To whom is the support provided? Who is providing the support? What kind of support is being provided? For which problem is support provided? What are the costs of giving and receiving support? How do these various issues interact in determining support level?" (pp. 10-11). More simply stated, who gives what to whom regarding which problem (House, 1981) and with what effect (Pearlin, 1985)? These queries implicitly reveal controversial concepts surrounding the disposition, duration, direction, and drawbacks of support that demand exploration by those interested in explicating its theoretical properties.

Disposition

Social support concepts can be operationally classified as social embeddedness, perceived social support, and enacted support. Social embeddedness refers to connections that individuals have to significant others in their social environment. Perceived social support is the cognitive appraisal of being reliably connected to others. Enacted support can be conceptualized as actions that others perform when they render assistance to individuals (Barrera, 1986; Tardy, 1985).

Perceived support refers to a generalized appraisal that individuals are "cared for and valued, that significant others are available to them in times of need, and that they are satisfied with the relationships they have" (Heller, Swindle, & Dusenbury, 1986). These esteem-enhancing appraisals of support stem from interactions (Thoits, 1986). Perceived social support reflects the information and feedback functions identified by Cobb (1976) and Cassel (1976). It influences how supportive transactions are interpreted, remembered, and associated with high self-esteem, low dysfunctional attitudes, and psychological distress (Lakey & Cassady, 1990). Low perceived support is associated with a tendency to perceive supportive attempts as unhelpful and to recall fewer instances of helpful supportive behavior.

Received support indicates what people get from others. It reflects the recipient's view of support reported to have come from others that was helpful or intended to be helpful (Sarason et al., 1990). *Enacted support* reflects the provider's view and may operate indirectly by influencing coping behavior or perception of support availability (Lakey & Heller, 1988). Hence, received support represents a "confounded picture of support availability, coping skills, and perceived severity of life stress" (Thoits, 1982).

Dunkel-Schetter and Bennett's (1990) detailed analysis verifies conceptual and operational distinctions between received and available support. Discrepancies between available (perceived) and received support are explained by inaccurate judgments regarding amount of support expected and quality of support delivered. Interpersonal skills of providers, coping behavior and self-esteem of recipients, and characteristics of social relationships and networks mediate the discrepancies (Dunkel-Schetter & Bennett, 1990). It is important to distinguish whether the psychological sense of support, or the actual expression and exchange of certain types of support, or both, influence outcomes (Gottlieb & Selby, 1989). Coyne and Bolger (1990) contest the assumption that perception of support is more beneficial than received support. Yet, perceived subjective appraisal or perceived adequacy of support was related to prediction of well-being (Procidano & Heller, 1983; Tardy, 1985; Vaux & Harrison, 1985), whereas enacted support had a small positive relationship to satisfaction (Barrera & Bacash, 1990).

In summary, social support may be perceived as potentially available from the social network or may be actually delivered and received. Both forms are important in the coping process. Thus instruments could emphasize equally, in the terminology used by Caplan (1981), subjective and objective support. Subjective measures tap psychological or cognitive appraisals of support (Cohen & Syme, 1985; Sarason et al., 1990). Nevertheless, it is important to assess use of support as well as perceived availability and to evaluate the extent to which aspects of actual social interaction correspond to perceptions of available support. Use is influenced by both individual and network variables. For example, the extent to which a single parent seeks and uses support may depend on perceptions of types and sources of help available, personal independence, satisfaction with support rendered in the past, and number of friends and family members accessible and willing to provide support.

> As a new single parent, Mary is receiving emotional and informational support from her friends and her mother; however, she perceives inadequate practical support with finances, housework, and job hunting. Furthermore, support that she anticipated would be available (perceived) from coworkers did not materialize (received).

Duration

Duration, which is an indirect measure of durability, can be analyzed by identifying the length of time a tie or relationship has existed or the stability of support over a prolonged period. The ability of providers to sustain support is critical in the case of chronically ill persons or those suffering long-term losses (Cohen & Syme, 1985; Hall & Wellman, 1985; House & Kahn, 1985).

Alterations in support are concomitant with life-course changes and transitions (Kahn & Antonucci, 1980; Kasl & Wells, 1985; Pearlin, 1985). Further, many stressful situations have different phases requiring different forms of support (Dimond, 1985) and can be categorized according to duration. Some stressors may require more long-term support than others. Social support exchanges vary over time and have short- and long-term effects on participants (Shumaker & Brownell, 1984). Thus, those whose initial role is helper may eventually assume the role of "helpee" and vice versa (Rook & Dooley, 1985). This is particularly true among kin and intimates, whose relationships are long-term (Clark, 1983). A final phenomenon relevant to duration of support is the nonmaterialization of expected social support, exemplified in Peters-Golden's (1982) study of patients with breast cancer.

In short, the evolving process of the interaction of stressors and support over time should be reflected more in the literature on social support. There is a need, for example, to examine the changes that take place in an individual's network (Bernard et al., 1990). Inclusion of duration in assessment tools seems desirable.

> Once 6 months had passed, Mary noticed that former neighbors, coworkers, and some friends did not contact her as often as they used to prior to her divorce. Only support from her mother and her best friend continued despite the changes in her life. Her links with her children were persistent, but not necessarily supportive.

Direction

It would seem that bidirectional support over time can prevent unpleasant feelings of indebtedness and dependence. The source of social support, however, may influence its direction. For example, professional support is typically unidirectional. In contrast, "directedness," a social-network concept, is defined as the amount of mutual sharing or reciprocity (Mitchell & Trickett, 1982), which entails both receiving and providing support.

As social support is both given and received, these two directions are measured in instruments as the conveyance and/or receipt of support. The social-psychological literature stresses the significance of reciprocity in social support. Reciprocity in relationships preserves self-esteem and prevents feelings of inadequacy and lack of control in recipients and feelings of burden and strain in providers (Albrecht & Adelman, 1987). In chronic stressful situations, therefore, the provider may need to be reassured of the value of her or his contribution (appraisal support) or of the recipient's continued caring and love (emotional support). New parents presumably would have more opportunities than the ill or aged to reciprocate in the future because of the time-limited nature of their "stressor."

> Mary's relationship with her children seems to be solely in the role of support provider—as it had been with her husband. Support was conveyed in one direction only. In contrast, her interactions with her widowed mother seem to be two-way. Her mother assists with babysitting her 4-year-old and inviting the family to dinner. Mary is able to reciprocate by driving her mother to shop for groceries and to church. Their love and caring over a lifetime of an intimate relationship is now more bidirectional than when Mary was a child.

Drawbacks and Benefits

Support from the network may have positive and negative elements (Brenner, Norwell, & Limacher, 1989; Fisher, Goff, Nadler, & Chinsky, 1988; Malone, 1988). Recognition that social support may have negative features is relatively recent in the social-psychological literature. Support provided may be perceived as unhelpful, particularly when it undermines self-esteem. Further, social networks may be strained and conflicted. Some ties with friends and families are sources of stress and conflict rather than support (Barrera, Sandler, & Ramsay, 1981; Chesler & Barbarin, 1984; Hall & Wellman, 1985; Shumaker & Brownell, 1984). On the other hand, stressors on a network member can be experienced vicariously by that person's friends (Chapman & Pancoast, 1985; Shinn, Lehmann, & Wong, 1984).

Benefits of seeking support are impressive. Benefits include cognitive and affective support, helping others by discussing the problem, practical assistance, improvement in emotional and physical state, enhanced level of functioning, supporter intervention, closer relationships with the supporter, and relational obligation. Benefits such as receiving emotional validation, advice, or direct tangible help, however, can be offset by risks. People cope differently with the risks of seeking support according to their relationship with the provider (Dakof & Taylor, 1990; Fisher et al., 1988; Goldsmith & Parks, 1990). People cope on their own by self-help to the extent that they do not perceive a situation as problematic, because of perceptions of a reference group. Esteem or appraisal support is perceived as helpful, particularly from intimates, but perceived as unhelpful when it is absent or misguided. Misguided or absent informational support from peers and professionals is considered detrimental. Advice often is given without an assessment of the problem and may be inappropriate or unappreciated (Eckenrode & Gore, 1990; La Gaipa, 1990; Wortman & Lehman, 1985). Avoidance can be one of the most unhelpful actions of friends. Expressing negative affect, disagreement with interpretations, discouraging expression of beliefs, withholding advice, isolating, and consuming material resources are types of "social dissupport" (Malone, 1988). Thus, sources of specific types of support are significant. It is unclear whether actions are rated as helpful and unhelpful from different sources because of their "frequency" or "salience" (Dakof & Taylor, 1990).

Drawbacks of support affect both support providers and support recipients. Kessler, McLeod, and Wethington (1985) found clear evidence that women were more burdened than men by the costs of caring. Overload, overexposure to chronic and acute stresses, overprotection, emotional involvement, and overcommitment might be involved (Coyne & Delongis, 1986; Kessler et al., 1985; La Gaipa, 1990). Providers may experience drainage of personal resources (such as time, energy, and emotional nurturance), "social contagion," social stress, or uncertainty about invading privacy or invalidating receiver perceptions (Albrecht & Adelman, 1987; Brickman et al., 1982; Eckenrode & Gore, 1981; La Gaipa, 1990). Although initial support may be skilled and helpful, burnout, frustration, helplessness, and emotional overinvolvement of providers can erode or erase initial helpful support.

Difficulties for the support recipient include hindered growth, feared lack of support in the future, cognitive distortion of social exchange, advice that constrains options, learned helplessness, incurred relational costs, diminished trust in times of diminished resources, and balancing strong and weak relationships (Albrecht & Adelman, 1987; La Gaipa, 1990). Support may negatively impact the recipient's self-esteem and sense of control (Fisher et al., 1988; Malone, 1988) due to anticipated negative attributions of providers, uncertainty about the interaction, or ineffective and inappropriate disclosure of personal weakness. Incongruent assumptions about the responsibility for cause and solution of a problem can lead to secondary victimization of recipients (Brickman et al., 1982, 1983). Embarrassment, fear of violation of confidentiality or of stigma, and reluctance to burden the supporter may impede support seeking (Goldsmith & Parks, 1990). The demand for equity also may limit support seeking. Inequitable relationships are psychologically costly (Fisher et al., 1988; Greenberg & Westcott, 1983). Yet even within equitable relationships, support efforts do not always meet needs of recipients (Coyne, Wortman, & Lehman, 1988). Rook and Pietromonaco (1987) report ineffective helping, excessive helping, negative regulation, and unpleasant interactions. Providers may offer support that is inappropriate or ill matched to the needs of the recipient; support offers may be misinterpreted or ineffectual; unqualified positive regard may yield inaccurate feedback; and there may be differing perceptions of social exchange.

Dunkel-Schetter and Bennett (1990) explain the discrepancy between perceived and received support in terms of the negative and positive features of support. Negative interactions are more predictive of depressed mood and poor emotional health than supportive interactions (House, Landis, & Umberson, 1988; Rook, 1990; Schuster, Kessler, & Aseltine, 1990). Most social relationships have supportive and negative elements because of increasing stressful obligations for reciprocity and conflicts (Rook, 1990). The negativity in intimate relationships is most significant (Rook, 1990; Schuster et al., 1990). However, negative interactions occur less frequently than supportive interactions (Sandler & Barrera, 1984). Hence, both supportive and negative aspects of relationships should be assessed at the same time.

Diverse terms have been used to conceptualize problematic social interactions such as social conflict, social network stressors, negative interactions, negative social support, and social strain. Rook (1990) defines social strain as "actions by a social network member that may cause the individual to experience adverse psychological or physiological reactions." Sources of social strain should be distinguished. "Negative support" however, may be an oxymoron. It could be more useful to construe negative interactions as interpersonal stress rather than lack of support (Coyne & Bulger, 1990; Shinn et al., 1984).

Conflicted support is a narrower concept than negative social relationships, as providers offer at least one positive form of support (Barrera & Bacash, 1990). Even successful intimate relationships involve some conflict between partners, including lapses or miscarried support efforts (Coyne et al., 1988; Sarason, Sarason, & Pierce, 1990) and failed support modes or functions (Eckenrode & Gore, 1990). Recurrent conflicts are created by participants' lack of awareness of their own or their partners' needs or their implicit demands (Sarason et al., 1990). Networks may fail to offer support when conflict exists about the appropriate level of support (Fisher et al., 1988).

Insufficient social-psychological research has been done on the negative effects of informal support systems. Most instruments disregard fluctuations in relationships (La Gaipa, 1990; Malone, 1988). Research is needed that investigates the synergistic effects (Rook, 1990; Schuster et al., 1990) and the beneficial and negative aspects of social support. Goldsmith and Parks (1990) suggest that the support process entails conflicting desires to reveal and withhold personal information. Problematic social relationships may lead to decreased access to helpful information and decreased self-esteem (Brenner et al., 1989).

The threat to self-esteem model assumes that aid experienced as self-threatening is costly to the recipient (Fisher et al., 1988; Fisher, Nadler, & Whitcher-Alagna, 1983). People with high mastery and high self-esteem receive more social support (Dunkel-Schetter & Skokan, 1990). Help is offered more frequently for visible, nonthreatening problems. People may avoid help from successful peers, illustrating social-comparison stress, which diminishes self-esteem. People with low self-esteem seek aid because of willingness to admit inadequacies (Fisher et al., 1988). Reactance theory (Brehm & Brehm, 1981) predicts that help that restricts freedom is psychologically costly (Gottlieb & Selby, 1989; Fisher et al., 1988). Coyne et al. (1988) discuss the reciprocal influences of negative interactions. There is a trade-off between reliance on others and privacy or freedom. La Gaipa (1990) cast the giving and receiving of support in terms of a dialectical conflict of independence and dependence. Past experience will influence help seeking from outside peers. Individuals who have an internal locus of control benefit more from support and seek support more (Lefcourt, Martin, & Saleh, 1984; Riley & Eckenrode, 1986). Thus, numerous theoretical interpretations are proffered regarding the complexities and conflicts of interpersonal relationships and their negative and positive features.

> Mary finds that some unwanted advice from her friends diminishes her sense of self-esteem and confidence in her new role as single parent. Further, she is beginning to feel indebted to her best friend, who has provided many kinds of support during this time of crisis and has been available throughout many ups and downs. In contrast, she also is experiencing feelings of burden associated with being the sole care provider for her children. She is reminded of the conflicts and tensions in her recently disintegrated intimate relationship with her former spouse.

Theoretical Interpretations of Social Support

Coping Theory

Lazarus and Folkman (1984) define coping as "constantly changing cognitive and behavioral efforts to manage specific external and/or internal demands that are appraised as taxing or exceeding the resources of the person." Coping is determined by the relationship between the person and the environment; it is a transactional process with problem-focused and emotion-focused functions (Folkman & Lazarus, 1980; Lazarus & Folkman, 1984).

Lazarus and Folkman (1984) treat social support under the rubric of coping as a resource available in the social environment (social network). People, they argue, must cultivate and may or may not call upon this social network, depending on access to alternative coping strategies. In addition, Lazarus and Folkman (1984) view social support as "a transactional process that changes with demands of the stressful encounter" and as a multidimensional construct, encompassing emotional, tangible, and informational functions. Thoits (1986) reconceptualized social support as coping assistance. Wells (1989) argues that support should be defined in terms of categories of coping.

Briefly, from a coping theorist's perspective, the perception of social support is one element in an individual's appraisal of the significance of a stressor for personal well-being (Procidano & Heller, 1983). Moreover, social support is one of a variety of potential coping resources (Gore, 1985; Sarason & Sarason, 1985; Tilden, 1985c). Social support, like other coping resources, regulates negative effects of stressful conditions. At times, it may be the only available coping method; at other times, it may not be either the most preferred or the most cost-effective method (Kasl & Wells, 1985).

Social support should be considered within the context of the stress and coping process, as socially mediated coping (Gottlieb, 1988a). Social networks and social support are more than resources to be called upon at will. In fact, social networks influence help seeking from formal and informal sources and attributions (appraisal) regarding causes and solutions for stressors, thereby influencing the coping process. Dunkel-Schetter, Folkman, and Lazarus (1987) purport that information is communicated to providers by coping strategies of recipients. Positive reappraisal lessens the threat of offering assistance. Moreover, social support and other cognitive and behavioral means of coping have reciprocal or bidirectional effects; the ways an individual copes provide important clues to potential supporters about whether support is needed and, if it is, about the types of support needed. Similarly, the receipt of support can later change the trajectory of coping.

Social support, like other coping resources, can modify the impact of chronically stressful conditions and acute stressors on health status (see Chapter 2). Gottlieb and Selby (1989) suggest that "examination of situational specific models of social support's effects will be more profitable than attempts to develop a grand theory that accounts for its impact on coping and health." Barbee, Gulley, and Cunningham (1990) propose a general model of interactive coping in which affect, cognition, and relationship and personal variables influence whether the coping strategies chosen pertain to dismissing or solving (problem-focused) or to escape or support (emotion-focused).

Silver, Wortman, and Crofton (1990) demonstrate that coping strategies influence type and quality of support received. People who use avoidance and distancing have fewer support resources (Billings & Moos, 1981). Problem solving, seeking support, and positive reappraisal were associated with greater support received. Support seeking is a specific coping behavior linked to greater provision of support (Dunkel-Schetter & Skokan, 1990). Yet, support-seeking behaviors may elicit or discourage giving needed support (Barbee, 1990). Dunkel-Schetter and Bennett (1990) suggest that the "nature and skill of a person's coping strategies applied to particular stressful situations may mediate the extent to which available support materializes." Coping portrayals can influence the course of the interaction and the nature and quality of support received (Silver et al., 1990). Individuals who present themselves as coping well generate positive responses but may not signal a need for support, leading to feelings of alienation and unrealistic expectations. Highlighting poor coping, however, may lead to denigration, rejection, or avoidance. A balanced self-presentation, in which disclosure of distress is accompanied by indications of coping efforts, positively influences support and appropriateness of type of support provided. Thus, social support influences coping abilities and coping strategies influence support sought and received; however, these reciprocal processes require further investigation.

> Mary is coping with her transition to single-parent status by seeking support from her own parent and best friend. She is reluctant to seek assistance, however, from more casual acquaintances, who do not seem to respond to her apparent inability to cope with unemployment.

Social Comparison Theory

People will make upward comparisons with those coping better than they are (who serve as role models) and downward comparisons to enhance self-esteem and protection (Taylor, 1983). Social comparison can be defined as people's tendency to evaluate themselves and to elicit information about their characteristics, behavior, opinions, and abilities through comparison with similar others. The basic tenet of Festinger's (1954) theory is that individuals evaluate themselves through social comparison with others to validate and define reality. Clearly, this evaluation process influences self-concept (Fisher & Nadler, 1982; Sanders, 1982; Suls, 1977; Wills, 1985).

The process of both upward and downward comparison occurs in mutual aid (groups) and, depending on the direction and dimension of comparison, will influence emotions, coping effectiveness, and prevention (Brickman et al., 1982; Gottlieb, 1985c; Shinn et al., 1984). The two types of comparisons are reference-group comparisons

(Merton, 1968) and person-other comparisons (Homans, 1961). Both are relevant to lay helpers.

Feedback from peers can provide validation and normalization (Chesler & Yoak, 1984). Comparison with others who are worse off diminished feelings of victimization among breast cancer patients and depressed subjects (Gottlieb & Selby, 1989; Wood, Taylor, & Lichtman, 1985). Nevertheless, social comparison with peers can negatively affect mental health through foreseeing a dismal future (Gottlieb & Selby, 1989), as in caregivers of seniors with Alzheimer's disease and people with multiple sclerosis.

Feedback from nonpeers, such as friends and family, can have positive effects (e.g., Coates & Winston, 1983; Gottlieb & Selby, 1989). Social support from a family is consistently sought throughout the life cycle (Horman, 1989). However, if the timing of major life transitions is atypical, individuals may experience negative social sanctions for deviating from norms, unflattering social comparison, fewer support resources (Rook, Catalano, & Dooley, 1989), and increased psychological distress.

Social comparison is a logical theoretical basis for determining whether people are similar in terms of health status, illness severity, stressor mastery, or coping stage (Gottlieb, 1988a). Health professionals, wishing to explain and evaluate positive and debilitating effects of peer helpers and mutual-aid groups on clients, should recall that upward comparison facilitates coping through modeling and downward comparison facilitates emotional adjustment in support dyads and groups. Certainly social comparison theory is relevant to the social support associated with target groups of health professionals, namely the bereaved, the ill, new parents, and the elderly. It is safe to assume that these people, like the cancer victims studied by Taylor (1983), would make upward comparisons with those coping better than they are for modeling purposes and downward comparisons to enhance self-esteem. The relevance of both social comparison and social exchange to social support is intuitively appealing because comparison by partners and exchange of resources occur in supportive relationships. Both theories can be used to interpret positive and negative reactions to help received from a peer.

> Responding to the advice of her best friend, Mary joined a support group for single mothers. She compares herself to other women, more experienced in this role, who seem to be coping more effectively than she is at present. However, she also

contrasts her situation to that of a woman who has been left with six young children and is receiving Social Security benefits. Thus she compares herself with her peers in two directions: upward regarding coping ability and downward in terms of severity of stressor.

Social Exchange Theory

Social exchange theory represents a merging of facets of social comparison (Festinger, 1954), cognitive dissonance (Festinger, 1954), and distributive justice (Rawls, 1971) theories. Social exchange constructs have been used implicitly as formulations by pioneer social support theorists in their descriptions of the reciprocal quality of support interactions (Caplan, 1974; Cobb, 1976). Similarly, Shumaker and Brownell's (1984) definitional phrase "exchange of resources" reaffirms these pioneering descriptions. Equity theories (Adams, 1963; Blau, 1964; Gouldner, 1960; Homans, 1961) suggest that a desire to maintain equity of exchanges exists in relations.

People may be unwilling to seek or accept help if they feel unable to return the benefit. For example, when aid is involuntary, relationships will be negatively influenced if actual or potential reciprocity does not exist (Chesler & Barbarin, 1984; DePaulo, 1982; Fisher et al., 1983; Gottlieb & Selby, 1989; Heller & Mansbach, 1984). The extent to which recipients feel indebted depends on their perception of the magnitude of rewards and costs incurred by both participants, the donor's motives, and cues from peers (Greenberg & Westcott, 1983; Shumaker & Brownell, 1984).

Norms of reciprocity and equity suggest, therefore, that support should be bidirectional. Reciprocity is the perception of bidirectional exchange of valued resources (Tilden & Galyen, 1987). Unfortunately, reciprocity is not always feasible. The physically and psychologically ill frequently encounter nonegalitarian and nonreciprocal relationships (DePaulo, 1982; Leavy, 1982; Wortman, 1984). Indeed, most network ties are asymmetric (Biegel & Naparstek, 1982).

As social exchange models suggest, support can involve benefits and costs for both recipients and providers. Costs are the perception of effort expended and debits incurred. Social interactions can have negative as well as positive effects on well-being. Perceptions of benefits or costs can affect perceptions of support availability and help seeking (Cohen & Syme, 1985; Shinn et al., 1984; Tilden &

Galyen, 1987). Measures can distinguish a person's experience as a support provider or a recipient (Dunkel-Schetter & Skoken, 1990).

A long-term relationship could allow members of a dyad to believe that reciprocity would be achieved eventually (Antonucci & Jackson, 1990). Clark (1984) distinguished communal, intimate relationships from exchange relationships where economic calculations are integral. In communal relations, concern about the other partner predominates (Perlman & Fehr, 1987). For people who are not in intimate relationships, reciprocity is expected more quickly and in kind. Intimates or kin may have developed a "bank of credits" (La Gaipa, 1990), a "support reserve" (Antonucci, 1985), or a "support bank" (Antonucci & Jackson, 1990). These persons may take a long-term developmental view of their social exchanges. Life-span reciprocity in longer-term relationships (Antonucci & Jackson, 1990; Clark & Reis, 1988) will influence the elderly's coping with declining resources. Gottlieb's (1989) analysis of family caregivers of the elderly suggests that the extent to which asymmetry of resources is perceived as chronologically equitable is more likely to affect the experience of subjective burden than the degree of actual equity achieved—by restoring equity for past or future benefits. Recipients may alleviate distress by reciprocity, but also by altering perceptions (Fisher et al., 1983).

Perceived reciprocity is an important ingredient in the impact of support. Reciprocal confiding relationships did not predict life satisfaction in Ingersoll-Dayton and Antonucci's (1988) study, although reciprocity with spouse was linked to life satisfaction by Kahn and Antonucci (1980). Support reciprocity was associated with diminished loneliness among widows (Rook, 1987) and highest well-being in self-help group members (Maton, 1987). Negative effects of inequity may depend on the type of relationship and the nature of support (La Gaipa, 1990).

Partners in equitable relationships are more likely to progress to higher levels of intimacy; to be content; to reestablish equity; and to persist in long-term, stable relationships (Hatfield & Sprecher, 1983; Perlman & Fehr, 1987). Conversely, asymmetry in the exchange of spousal support may limit willingness to offer support (Eckenrode & Gore, 1990). Support providers who are not rewarded by appreciation and signs of improvement may stop trying to help (Dunkel-Schetter & Bennett, 1990).

Mutual caring, important to social support, can be trivialized by cost-benefit analysis. An equity model focuses on negative reactions to support (Fisher et al., 1983). The process of giving and receiving help is more "fluid" and long-term than implied by exchange theories (Antonucci & Jackson, 1990).

> Mary gradually discovers that she is exchanging ideas regarding coping strategies, community resources, and job opportunities, and is sharing child-care responsibilities with other mothers in her support group. Furthermore, she encourages her teenage daughter to assist with the housework and to contribute money earned in babysitting to the household finances. Mary, in turn, continues to enact her role as mother and key support provider for Shelley.

Attribution Theory

When individuals assign blame for the origin of a problem and ascribe control over the problem to either the provider or the recipient, this influences helping relationships. Attributions blaming the recipient for failure or negative motives of the provider are threatening (Brickman et al., 1982; Fisher et al., 1983, 1988). In contrast, attributions that render the problem soluble, if help is sought, and diminish self-threat enable help seeking. The search for meaning and mastery in threatening events is attributional (Taylor, 1983). Attribution theory (Heider, 1958; Kelley, 1967) posits that individuals will formulate attributions to understand, predict, and control their environment according to relative weights assigned to internal (person) or external (environment) factors.

Explanations of responsibility for causing and solving a person's problems have been used to construct four discrete helping models. The compensatory, enlightenment, medical, and moral models are delineated by Brickman et al. (1982, 1983). According to these unique conceptualizations of helping, responsibility for causing or solving a problem can be attributed by potential help-givers to the individuals rather than the environment. These models can interpret health professionals' views of client problems, as professionals may assign to the client blame for the cause or responsibility for solution. Furthermore, assessment of attributions can explain the perceptions and motives of help-seekers and of lay helpers. In this context, Ryan (1985) applied attribution theory to compare and explain the different helping models preferred by different lay support groups and professionals.

Perceptions of responsibility for a problem should increase one's sense of personal responsibility to help. Caregivers' attributions reflect their perceptions of the legitimacy of the recipients' needs and of their deservingness of support. Social support can foster attribution of personal control and of self-esteem if problems are attributed to factors beyond the recipient's control (Gottlieb & Selby, 1989), and attributions can in turn enhance understanding of relationships (Baucom, 1987). Baucom (1987) portrays an apparent relationship between marital adjustment and attributions of the partners. According to Gottlieb (1988a), "there is moot evidence about the effect that these causal and control attributions have on affect, behavior and self perception." However, the attribution-affect-action link may be particularly strong for practical support offered to strangers (Dunkel-Schetter & Skokan, 1990). Although impact on behavior is unclear, persons' attributions and perceptions affect support preferred and sought.

> Some of Mary's more casual friends found it easy to blame her for her recent misfortunes. Why didn't she stay with her husband, who was secure financially? She must have done something wrong to lose him to a younger woman. Therefore she should be responsible for solving her own problems. Not surprisingly, little support was forthcoming from these persons. The support group, in contrast, attributed the cause of Mary's problems to external factors beyond her control and were willing to share some of the responsibility of helping her look for solutions.

Social Learning Theory

Social learning theory posits that people's perception of their capabilities affects their behavior, thinking, and emotional reactions in stressful situations (O'Leary, 1985). Further, it postulates that personal and situational influences alter coping behavior and transactions with the social environment (Bandura, Reese, & Adams, 1982; Mowrer, 1960). Developed by Bandura (1977), social learning theory successfully synthesizes cognitive, behavioral, emotional, and environmental explanations of learning and behavioral changes.

Self-efficacy theory, developed within the framework of social learning theory, concerns the effects of self-referent thought on psychosocial functioning (O'Leary, 1985). Self-efficacy is one's belief that one can perform some behavior or use some cognitive strategy to meet the demands of a given situation. Self-knowledge about personal efficacy is based on four principal sources of information: performance attainment or skills mastery, vicarious observation of others' performance, verbal persuasion and other forms of social influence, and reinterpretation of physiological status (Gonzales, Goepperinger, & Lorig, 1990). However, according to Bandura (1986), most human behavior is developed by modeling.

Role modeling, a primary concept of social learning theory, is an important component of helping relationships. Peers have available a range of stress coping, behavior change, and mastery models. Modeling has been described in studies of self-help groups for new mothers (Unger & Wandersman, 1985), for anorexia nervosa and bulimia victims (Kinoy, 1985), for child abusers (Wodarski, 1981), for low-income African-American and Hispanic families (Maida, 1985), for stroke survivors (Banks, 1985), and for cardiovascular patients (Levy, 1983).

According to a theoretical framework created by Borkman (1976), peers, viewed as role models, elicit and enhance experiential knowledge. Experiential knowledge, specialized information of a phenomenon based on firsthand experience, is developed within self-help groups. This type of wisdom is concrete, specific, pragmatic, holistic, and oriented to here-and-now action. Self-help groups develop, disseminate, and validate this type of knowledge, which can be distinguished from information relayed by professionals. People can assimilate new knowledge better when it is presented by peers because they can identify with someone who shares a common experience. Experiential knowledge facilitates the cathartic and empathetic dimensions in mutual-aid groups (Silverman, 1980).

Katz (1985) comments that "though Borkman does not use their terminology, her descriptions parallel the concepts of role modeling and reinforcement advanced by . . . social learning theorists." Other references to social learning theory in the support literature are minimal. Silverman (1980) noted that learning can be enhanced in a peer context, and Maida (1985) applied social learning theory to analyze an approach used to reinforce new role experiences in self-help groups. Likewise, Bandura (1986), the prolific social learning theorist, has only begun to acknowledge the significance of social support. He claims that "personal change occurs within a network of social influences . . . development of longer term social support for beneficial styles of behavior."

Several social learning concepts may be particularly germane to mutual-aid groups and lay helpers: reciprocal determinism, vicarious experiences (including role modeling previously described), social persuasion, collective comparison, and self- and collective efficacy (Stewart, 1990b). Bandura's social learning theory is a general theory of behavior that can be used to interpret behavior change and cognitive change mechanisms in support dyads and groups. Social learning theory may explain empowerment and personal control, germane to social competence.

> Within the support group, role modeling by women who had successfully dealt with similar problems taught Mary alternative coping strategies and raised her personal sense of capability (efficacy). She felt empowered to pursue different types of employment opportunities. Furthermore, the group worked collectively to effect changes in the town's financial support of single parents and in the provision of child care by potential employers.

Social Competence

Social support has been viewed as an outcome of social competence (Broadhead et al., 1983). Theoretical knowledge of social support processes may be a component of relational competence (Hobfoll & Freedy, 1990). Dispositional variables of recipients include social skills (Heller et al., 1986; Sarason, Sarason, Hacker, & Basham, 1985). Competence and skills may cause people to establish and maintain social relationships and may affect their quality (House, Landis, & Umberson, 1988). The social competence skills necessary for forming and maintaining relationships, including social problem-solving skills, empathy, and comfort in intimate relationships, are qualities of a self-actualizing person (Ford & Procidano, 1990). People who are low in perceived social support have poorer social skills and are not able to initiate or maintain relationships or communicate their needs (Barbee, Gulley, & Cunningham, 1990). Unassertive caregivers typically have less available social support (Robinson, 1990), indicating that social skills are an important antecedent of available social support. Mastery and self-esteem also are important in soliciting support.

The sense of "perceived competence" is likely to have a critical influence on whether experience as either a provider or a recipient leads to increased support efforts (Dunkel-Schetter & Skokan, 1990). Subjects with high social competence scored higher in terms of received and perceived social support (Sarason et al., 1985). Competence-promoting support is developed in the context of low network strain (Tucker & Johnson, 1989).

Gottlieb and Selby (1989) speculate on the possibility of social competence interventions optimizing support receipt. The lonely may not only seek less support but also lack the necessary social or communication skills to initiate and maintain relationships, and they may have difficulty with sharing and self-disclosure. Social skills training has met with some success (Adelman, Parks, & Albrecht, 1987; Hobfoll & Freedy, 1990; Jones, 1985).

> Mary has learned how to approach others and to seek support appropriately from people within and outside the support group. She and her children gradually have enhanced their social skills to develop new friendships and contacts. Sean has had to learn to accommodate his speech handicap in his attempts to communicate with the children of the other women in the group. This competence, in turn, has diminished the family's sense of isolation and loneliness following the move.

Summary

Attribution theory can enable explanation of donors' motives, the phenomena of help seeking and helping, and the possible negative effects of support efforts. Coping theory demonstrates how social support and coping interface in the stress process by acknowledging individual and environmental perspectives, adds a cognitive dimension to support, and considers costs of support efforts. Equity theory explains reactions to support from donor and recipient viewpoints, the reciprocal nature of social support, its impact on help seeking, and its beneficial and detrimental features. Social comparison theory is helpful in interpreting and evaluating positive and debilitating effects of support when the donor is a peer. Social learning and self-efficacy theory enables explanation of influences on persons' coping, behavior, and transactions with the social environment. Self-efficacy, in turn, is linked to social competence.

Regrettably, explicit conceptual linkages are not delineated in Gonzalez, Goepperinger, and Lorig's (1990) study of self-efficacy, coping, and social support theory in patient education or in any other published research.

Measurement of the Construct

Network properties that are amenable to measurement include size (number of people in the focal unit), homogeneity (the similarity of persons in the network), reciprocity (the degree of support given and received), duration (changes in the network over time), multiplexity (the extent of multiple communication contents in the link), and density (interconnections of contacts) (Albrecht & Adelman, 1987; House & Kahn, 1985). Objective measures of properties of networks, such as number of members, provide estimates of embeddedness in society. However, size is only weakly linked to availability or adequacy of support. Furthermore, network analyses have not proven their usefulness in the study of social support's relationship to health outcomes (Sarason et al., 1990). Functional measures should predict health outcomes better than these structural measures (Cohen & Syme, 1985).

Some measures examine availability of support; others examine its enactment. Support availability refers to quantity or quality of support to which people have access, whereas the actual use of these support resources is enacted support. Other measures assess frequency of helping behaviors or actions involved in assistance (Barrera, 1986; Tardy, 1985).

Support perceived as available can only be described, but support actually received can be described and/or evaluated. Evaluation measures individuals' satisfaction with social support, whereas descriptive instruments only portray type and source of social support. Some measures of perceived support emphasize availability and others stress satisfaction (Popiel & Susskind, 1985; Sarason et al., 1990; Wellman, 1985). Qualitative measures of social support are considered by some (e.g., Griffith, 1985) to be superior because of their greater predictive power regarding personal adjustment. This may be because a perceived sense of social support derives from subjective estimates of adequacy of support (Gottlieb, 1985b).

Extant measures focus on either received or perceived support, as exemplified in Table 1.2. Most measures of social support assess

(text continued on page 32)

Table 1.2 Selected Social-Support Instruments

Instrument	*Perceived or Received Measures*	*Items*	*Responses*
Arizona Social Support Interview Schedule	Received support	# of people available for 6 types of interactions (confiding, material aid, advice, positive feedback, physical assistance, social participation)	How many people actually provided each function in past month
CCISS (Bennett, Gottlieb, & Cadman, 1987)	Received support	Support received within a particular population, caregivers of children with chronic illness (emotional, appraisal, instrumental, informational)	
Interpersonal Support Evaluation List (Cohen et al., 1985)	Perceived/available support (perceived availability of potential social resources)	48 items; 4 subscales: —appraisal —belonging —tangible —self-esteem	4-part response: —strongly agree —disagree
Inventory of Socially Supportive Behaviors (Barrera et al., 1981, 1984)	Received support	40 specific supportive behaviors represent 4 types: —emotional —tangible —cognitive/informational —directive guidance	
Life Stressors and Social Resources Inventory (Moos et al., 1988)	Received support	Taps stable and new aspects of life stressors and social resources in 8 domains: physical health, home/neighborhood, financial, work, spouse/partner, children, extended family, and friends	Questions tap potentially helpful conditions or aspects of relationships

Moos Family Environment Scale	Perceived/available support	10 subscales of 9 items each covering 3 dimensions —family relations —family growth —family maintenance	
Multidimensional Scale of Perceived Social Support (Dahlem et al., 1991)	Perceived/available support	12 item ratings	7-pt. Likert scale, very stongly disagree to very strongly agree
Perceived Social Support	Perceived/available support (perceived from family or friends)	20 items	yes/no/don't know
Social Network and Support Interview Tool (Moxley, 1988)	Received/available support; perceived emotional support	Interview questions assessing network size and structure, duration, frequency of contact, and perceived emotional relationships	Contacts within the last 3 months
Social Support Questionnaire (Sarason et al., 1983)	Perceived/available support	27 different situations 2 scores —average # of available support providers —average level of satisfaction with available support	Past sources; each situation rate satisfaction
Stress Questionnaire (Dunkel-Schetter, Folkman, & Lazarus, 1987)	Received support	Specific support received from specific sources in context of specific stressful episodes (information, aid, emotional)	

respondents' sense of quality or adequacy of social support rather than their actual receipt of support. Measures can distinguish perceptions of recipients and providers (Dunkel-Schetter & Skokan, 1990). The proliferation of these and other social support measures is evident in reviews by Gottlieb and Selby (1989), House and Kahn (1985), O'Reilly (1988), Popiel and Susskind (1985), and Tardy (1985).

There has been insufficient psychometric evaluation or attention to construct validity (House & Kahn, 1985; Tardy, 1985; Weinert & Tilden, 1990). Measurement difficulties arise because of the multifaceted nature of the construct and lack of consensus of how to measure it. Most measures do not gather information about the support process or the interaction or communication of social support. Some measures fail to differentiate social embeddedness, perceived social support, and enacted support (Barrera, 1986; Gottlieb & Selby, 1989). No measures of social support have been designed for different ethnic groups or cultures. However, measures recently have been administered to children (Gottlieb & Selby, 1989). Specific or situation-specific measures are emerging that refer to groups of stressed subjects facing common crisis and also examine specific types and sources of social support as well as satisfaction with received support (Popiel & Susskind, 1985). The level of specificity of measurement of stressors, receipt of support, and well-being (Dunkel-Schetter & Bennett, 1990) should be comparable.

There is a need to assess the context of supportive transactions and to go beyond individual self-reports of perceived support to observe how relationships influence adaptation (Coyne & Bolger, 1990). Evidence indicates that qualitative features such as conflict, overinvolvement, or ambivalence are related more strongly to well-being (Pierce et al., 1990). Social support measures therefore should distinguish between network members who provide only positive forms of social support and those who are sources of negative interaction (Barrera et al., 1981) and should examine the "overall balance of sustaining and discordant influences" (Gottlieb, 1983, p. 62).

Summary

The construct of social support has been conceptualized in diverse definitions from varying perspectives of sociologists, anthropologists, epidemiologists, and psychologists. Distinctions between social networks and social support are made in structural and functional approaches, respectively. Some of these distinctions can be explained by the fact that support may be perceived or received, may vary in stability and duration, may be unidirectional or bidirectional, and may have both negative and positive features. A variety of theories—coping, social comparison, social exchange, attribution, social learning, and social competence—can be invoked to interpret these distinct dimensions. Furthermore, these dimensions and distinctions can be measured to yield operational definitions of the construct.

❖ CHAPTER TWO ❖

Social Support
Impact on Health, Health Behavior, and Health Care

Relevance of Social Support to Health Professionals

Social support should be of particular interest to health professionals because of its impact on health, health behavior, and health-services utilization. Reviews (Broadhead et al., 1983; Brownell & Shumaker, 1985; Cohen & Syme, 1985; Cohen & Wills, 1985) indicate that social support has direct, indirect, and interactive effects on physical and mental health. Berkman (1985) postulates that lay networks exert peer pressure on health behavior or lifestyle-related activities practiced through individual choice. Further, as noted in Chapter 1, social networks influence help seeking from health professionals and complement or even replace professional services (Whittaker & Garbarino, 1983). Informal networks can convert lay needs into resources. As Tilden (1985c) declares, the power of informal support lies in its omnipresence, its locus of control within persons, and its cost-effectiveness.

Impact of Support on Health: Competing Explanations

Integration in a network and the ability to draw resources from the network can maintain health and facilitate physical recovery (Bloom, 1990; Caplan, 1974). Kaplan and Toshima (1990) review evidence that social support enhances health outcomes and reduces mortality, whereas poor, stressful social relationships can prolong physical dysfunction. Epidemiological studies link social network to morbidity and mortality—the socially integrated are less likely to have high rates of tuberculosis, depression, hypertension, accidents, pregnancy complications, and schizophrenia (Ford & Procidano, 1990; House, Landis, & Umberson, 1988; Minkler, 1986; Sullivan & Poertner, 1989)—but do not explain why social relationships enhance health. Current research focuses on three hypotheses: Social support may prevent stress; social support buffers or cushions stress; and social support may have a direct positive effect on health unrelated to stress (Tilden & Weinert, 1987).

Main, Moderating, and Mediating Effects

The *main-effect model* proposes that social support directly benefits well-being by fulfilling basic social needs (Thoits, 1982) and enhancing social integration (Cohen & Wills, 1985). The main effect is equivalent to a primary preventive function and is explained in part by social inoculation theory (Pilisuk, 1982), which posits that social support has "been shown experimentally to influence susceptibility to some infections, to some neoplastic processes, and to some aspects of the humoral and cell mediated immune response" (p. 23). Integration in a social network could be related to physical health outcomes through emotionally induced effects on neuroendocrine or immune system functioning (Cohen & Wills, 1985). Conversely, disruptive life events can rend social networks and may thereby suppress the immune system (Gottlieb, 1987).

The *buffering model* posits that support protects individuals from potentially harmful influences of acute stressful events and enhances coping abilities. Three pioneer authors of theoretical papers on social support supported Cassel's (1974) premise that psychosocial stressors "will, by altering the endocrine balance in the body, increase the susceptibility of the organism to . . . disease agents" (p. 473). Caplan

(1974, p. 3) endorsed Cassel's suggestion that the most significant buffering, cushioning processes were available primary-group supports. Cobb (1976) claims that these supports could "protect people in crisis from a wide variety of pathological states" (p. 310). Okun, Sandler, and Baumann (1988) explain that the buffer effect of social support reduces the negative impact of negative life events, while the booster effect enhances the beneficial impact of positive life events. Their research with college students provided evidence for both effects. Thus, under certain circumstances, social support may cushion the impact of stressful life events and amplify the beneficial effect of positive life events. Thoits (1986) queries, however, whether life events are distressing because they demand readjustment in daily patterns or because they deprive the individual of important support resources. Social support around events can enhance coping by meeting needs generated or by appraising the event as less likely to have harmful consequences (Cohen & Wills, 1985; Okun et al., 1988). The buffering hypothesis assumes that individuals with strong support should be better able to cope with major life changes (Cohen & Syme, 1985; Thoits, 1986). Social support may be a primary coping resource or may interact with the coping response to affect level of stress (Bloom, 1990).

Contextual factors such as social support and coping resources are considered moderators. Quittner, Gluechauf, and Jackson (1990) indicate that the moderator model and the buffer model are similar. The moderator model predicts that perceived social support interacts with stress level to modify psychological adjustment; hence, social support is perceived to be most beneficial under conditions of high stress.

The mediator model predicts that social support acts as an intervening variable indirectly influencing the effects of stress on health (Quittner et al., 1990). For example, parents reporting chronic burden might experience reduced social interaction through role loss, drained resources, conflicted social interaction, or unwanted support, which in turn would be associated with poorer mental health status. Eckenrode and Gore (1990) differentiate stress-mediating processes that involve the pathways through which stress impacts on well-being and stress-moderating processes that prevent stress from crossing over from one role or person to the next or that determine reactivity to stress.

Research testing these three effects of social support uses different methodologies and reports inconsistent results. Studies of functions or types of support usually find evidence of buffering effects and studies of social integration find main effects (Cohen & Wills, 1985). However, most researchers have focused upon buffering effects and have failed to examine the "theoretically and practically significant" main effects of social support on stress (Thoits, 1982). Different mechanisms or processes are behind each (Heller et al., 1986; Thoits, 1986). The two concepts are likely to be least convergent under conditions of high stress (Dunkel-Schetter & Bennett, 1990). Schwarzer and Leppin's (1989) review of 55 studies "endorse[s] the assumption that social support is related to health conditions, especially for women and in stress situations" (p. 10). In contrast, Vaux (1990) contends that support and stressors are not independent, as assumed in tests of the buffering hypothesis, but can only be understood within an ecological context.

Support for main versus buffering models involves testing the interaction between social support and life events; absence of interaction favors the main-effect model and presence of interaction favors the stress-buffering effect. Empirical evidence has been mixed (Landerman, George, Campbell, & Blazer, 1989). Life events exerted stronger effects on depressive outcomes when there was inadequate support (consistent with the stress-buffering hypothesis). It is not clear how social embeddedness protects health or how receipt of social support exerts its moderating or buffering impact on stressful life events. Prospective mortality studies find social relationships associated inversely with mortality (Berkman & Syme, 1979; Blazer, 1982; House, Landis, & Umberson, 1988; House, Robbins, & Metzner, 1982). These studies found a curvilinear association and a nonspecific physical health impact. Cohen and Wills (1985) note that buffering effects emerge with measures of perceived availability of functional support or when specific types of support are matched to specific stressors, whereas main effects emerge with broad, structured social-network measures and measures of social integration's effect on stability and self-esteem.

The distinction between received and perceived support (introduced in Chapter 1) illuminates some of the differences in effects. Perception of available support, unlike received support, moderates the relationship between stress and psychological outcomes (Cohen, Mermelstein, Kamarck, & Hoberman, 1985; Wethington & Kessler, 1986). However, perceptions that support is available also may have a main effect on health because of a cognitive or psychological pathway

(Gottlieb, 1988a; Heller et al., 1986). The perception of available support reduced vulnerability to different stress-related disorders and influenced the outcome and course of illness (Cohen & McKay, 1984; Holohan & Moos, 1982; Kaplan et al., 1977; Soloman, Waysman, & Mikulincer, 1990). Soloman et al. (1990) concluded that perceived support did not have a direct protective effect, but rather promoted mental health through its impact on loneliness. Dunkel-Schetter and Bennett (1990) argue that received support, in terms of specific stressful situations and the support-activation process, should be considered in tests of buffer effects. Specificity models (Cohen & McKay, 1984; Thoits, 1986) assume that different stressful events require different coping strategies and support resources. Thus, Cohen and Wills (1985) found buffering effects for tangible assistance only when the stress entailed a loss of tangible assets. Further, emotional support has been linked to psychological outcomes and social integration to physical role functioning (Bloom, 1990).

In summary, four points intersect support and health. Two are stress buffering, one intervening from stressors-to-distress and the other intervening from distress-to-health outcomes. Social support's buffering role is in its influence on primary and secondary appraisal in the coping process. The other two junctions are direct or primary preventive: Social support may act as a well-being factor directly influencing morale and self-esteem (Barrera, 1986; Gottlieb & Selby, 1989). The appropriate research question now is not whether buffering/moderating, mediating, or main effects exist, but how these effects of support on health occur through a variety of processes or mechanisms.

Mechanisms Through Which Support Acts With Health

It remains unclear exactly how support may affect health, be it by behavioral or by physiological and biochemical pathways (Schwarzer & Leppin, 1989). Growing evidence indicates that support affects health; however, the physiological mechanisms are not well understood. Longitudinal and psychophysiological studies are needed to inform the causal process through which support influences health (Bloom, 1990), to trace mechanisms (Gottlieb & Selby, 1989; Pugliesi, 1989), and to follow at-risk populations (Kennedy, Kiecolt-Glaser, & Glaser, 1990). These mechanisms may be immunological, environmental, or bidirectional between health and the network.

Immunological

Clearly, the general social-support literature, although acknowledging the direct effects of support on health, has merely started to consider the potential relationship of social support and immunity to disease. Recent findings in the field of psychoneuroimmunology, on which the study of AIDS has focused public attention, could prove relevant.

Psychoneuroimmunology is a rapidly expanding field that encompasses behavioral sciences, neuroendocrinology, and immunology (Cunningham, 1981) and is concerned with the complex bidirectional interactions between the central nervous system and the immune system. This interaction appears to play a part in psychosocial influences on immunologically resisted and mediated illness (Solomon, 1987). Solomon and Amkraut (1981) assert that "Psychoneuroimmunological concepts began with clinical observations on the relationships of emotions to resistance to disease" (p. 157).

The immune system operates to protect the individual against invasion by foreign substances or organisms (Cunningham, 1981). "Immunological competence" is the capacity to identify and reject material foreign to the individual (Palmblad, 1981) and reflects the degree to which the organism is protected (Maeir, Landenslager, & Ryan, 1985). There is growing support for the view that psychosocial stress can have immunosuppressive effects (Darko, 1986).

Of particular potential interest to health professionals are the psychoneuroimmunological studies examining the impact of one stressor that involves depletion of the social network, specifically bereavement. These studies, conducted on healthy people, demonstrated that bereavement, with its accompanying emotional reactions, is associated with gradual depression in cell-mediated immunity. Bereaved individuals have a decrease in natural killer-cell activity (Darko, 1986). The psychoneuroimmunological literature refers to the possibility that certain kinds of tumors appear following bereavement (Palmblad, 1981) and to excess appearance of disease within the first year after this type of loss (Fox, 1981).

Loss of a significant love relationship through bereavement and other causes has been documented as preceding the onset of systemic lupus erythematosus (Solomon, 1981), ulcerative colitis, rheumatoid arthritis, leukemia (Gottschalk, 1983), and tumors (Solomon & Amkraut, 1981). Most children with juvenile rheumatoid arthritis have experienced network losses through parental divorce, separation, or death (Solomon, 1981). Poor marital quality and separation are associated with reduction in several measures of immune function and, in turn, with increased depression (Solomon, 1987). Fragmented or narrow social networks and deficient communication with others increase proneness to depressive disorders, poorer recovery from surgery, alcohol and drug abuse, and prolonged labor (Gottschalk, 1983). Conversely, depression has been found to be associated with lowered immune functioning. Thus a feedback loop may exist between depression and immune functioning.

Data from recent studies reveal that loneliness is associated with poorer immune function (Glaser, Kiecolt-Glaser, Speicher, & Holliday, 1985; Kennedy et al., 1990). Life situations characterized by alienation and social isolation have been associated with respiratory infections (Palmblad, 1981) and arthritis (Soloman, 1981). Kiecolt-Glaser et al. (1984) found that persons who had high loneliness scores had significantly lower levels of natural killer(NK)-cell activity and poorer T-lymphocyte responses to phytohemagglutin (presumably reflecting weaker cellular immune systems) than those who had low scores. In a slightly different context, Solomon noted that family caregivers of victims of Alzheimer's disease had reduced helper T-cell ratios and lower immune control of latent Epstein-Barr virus. Thus, support donors may experience stress that has negative immunological consequences.

Health-related changes following marital disruption may have an impact on the immune function (Kennedy et al., 1990). A marital relationship may simultaneously be a source of stress and impede seeking other support (Coyne & Delongis, 1986). Levy et al. (1990) confirmed the association between lower activity of NK cells and perception of poor quality of social support within the family. A striking association existed between the perception of positive quality of social support from spouse, family, and professionals and higher level of NK cell activity—thus perceived support predicted changes in NK cell activity and played a buffering role (Levy et al., 1990).

Knowledge about the supportive provisions or behaviors that increase immunity to illness or foster improved coping is required. For example, self-disclosure of traumatic events is associated with better immune function and physical health (Kennedy et al., 1990; Pennebaker, Kiecolt-Glaser, & Glaser, 1988). Writing about traumatic experience had positive effects on the blastogenic response of T-lymphocytes to mitogens and on autonomic levels. House (1981), a major contributor to the social support literature, however, legitimately contends that it is a "big step . . . from understanding how natural immunity works to intentionally and artificially synthesizing or enhancing the elements of such immunity" (p. 89).

Clearly, the intricate interrelationship of stress, diverse forms of support, and the immune system merit further exploration. Speculation regarding how stress affects immunocompetence continues. There appears to be agreement that stress activates both antuitary and opiate systems (Maier et al., 1985) via central nervous system and neuroendocrine mediation (Solomon, 1981). The hypothalamus may have a direct role (Solomon & Amkraut, 1981). Stressor exposure may depress a person's defense, as long as it prevails, or only for the initial phase of stress; a period of enhanced resistance may follow (Palmbald, 1981). Thus, diverse pathways have been proposed. However, psychoneuroimmunological studies often ignore the possibility that stress may lead to health behavioral changes that themselves may impair immunity and increase susceptibility to illness or infection. The outcome of these debates is potentially relevant to social support research.

Social Environment and Type of Relationship Within Social Network

Social environments influence health behavior and risks. Yet, there has been insufficient research into differences in disease rates in different social environments—research that could enhance disease prevention (Syme, 1987). Interventions may modify the social setting to minimize environmental stressors and to enhance appropriate support resources and behaviors.

Hall and Wellman (1985) suggest that the composition, structure, and content of interpersonal ties in social environments can be related to "the study of stress, social support and other health care issues" (p. 25). Density, reciprocity, and homogeneity appear to have the greatest impact on health and well-being (House & Kahn, 1985; House, Landis, & Umberson, 1988; Sarason et al., 1990; Seeman & Berkman, 1988). Reciprocity or bidirectional relationships have been found to be relevant to health and health promotion (e.g., House &

Kahn, 1985; House, Landis, & Umberson, 1988; Shinn et al., 1984; Tardy, 1985; Tilden & Galyen, 1987; Vaux & Athanassopulou, 1987). Conversely, nonsupportive or negative relationships increase the possibility of poor health (Antonucci, 1985; Berkman & Syme, 1979). Brenner et al. (1989) found that the presence of at least one source of consistently problematic interactions contributed significantly to less life satisfaction, and many sources of supportive interaction were also sources of problematic interactions. Problematic social ties exert negative effects on well-being (Rook, 1984).

According to the Functional Effects Model, the social environment can affect health outcomes, and, conversely, illness modifies the support environment. Some studies found that overconcern or nonsupportive behavior can be detrimental for health outcomes and self-care in diabetes, coronary heart disease, and asthma (Kaplan & Toshima, 1990).

Perlman and Fehr (1987) conclude that married persons have better health and well-being than nonmarried persons. Close, intimate, satisfying relationships have an impact on psychological health and mortality (Reiss, 1984). In fact, increased morbidity has been demonstrated in the absence of an intimate, confiding, close, intense relationship (Brown & Bifulco, 1985; Kobasa, Muddi, Puccetti, & Zola, 1985; Lefcourt, Martin, & Saleh, 1984). Supportive interactions and confidants may promote pain tolerance (Kaplan & Toshima, 1990). However, Pugliesi (1989) discovered that parenthood, not marital status or intimate contacts, had a positive effect on social participation and self-esteem. Marital status affected well-being directly when social support was controlled. Pugliesi's results did not support the contention that social roles affect levels of social support. It may be that individuals with greater self-confidence and well-being establish more social ties (Dooley, 1985) and role involvement in the social environment.

Impact of Illness on Network

Illness can be a major stressor involving loss of social mobility, loss of capacity to work, threat of death for the victim and for his or her intimates, loss of a loved one, loss of status or relationship, and loss of independence due to need for caregiving. The continued need for social support in chronic stress situations, such as illness, depletes the positive contribution of support and drains the resources that contribute to support. Furthermore, chronic illness may produce alienation and estrangement from the network.

Dunkel-Schetter and Wortman (1985) posit that victimizing events, such as cancer, can create conflicting reactions among network members. Wortman (1984), Wortman and Conway (1985), and Wortman and Lehman (1985) delineated the strained relationships; insensitive, uncaring behavior; and avoidance to which the physically ill are frequently subjected.

Lack of reciprocity characterizes relationships in which one person is gravely ill (Wortman & Conway, 1985). The impaired elderly report feelings of dependence and interpersonal difficulties with caregiving relatives (Parmalee, 1983). This suggests that the acutely and chronically ill experience nonreciprocal relationships with their social networks and with health professionals. Chronic physical illness points to the advisability of acknowledging provision of social support more explicitly, in conjunction with receipt of support. Surely the ill would have enhanced self-esteem and security in the relationship if they were enabled to offer certain types of support. Support would not necessarily have to be in kind. Jung (1990) found that familial reciprocity was more strongly associated with lowered symptoms than the amount of support either received or provided. He suggests that lack of reciprocity may be the result rather than the cause of high stress or illness symptoms.

The Conservation Of Resources Model posits that providing support drains resources (Hobfoll & Stevens, 1990a). Yet little attention has been paid to social networks or support as dependent variables (House, Kessler, & Herzog, 1990) in the interaction with health status.

> Mary develops a severe case of viral pneumonia one month after the move. Her recent loss through marital separation may have generated immunological changes so that she was less resistant to infection. Her recovery is delayed by recurrent exacerbations. Her mother is called upon to help care for the children, in addition to caring for her daughter. Over time this burden becomes too great, and her mother suffers exhaustion and illness. Mary does not have the physical strength to maintain her social contacts with her casual friends. Her illness has a deteriorating

effect on her network, but, conversely, her network loss may have provoked this illness.

Influence of Social Support on Health Behavior

The social network may influence health status outcomes directly through information or motivation for health behavior or indirectly through encouragement to comply with regimes or maintain health-promoting behavior such as exercise. Network members provide advice and models of behavior and extend support provisions that augment immunity (Bloom, 1990; Cohen & Wills, 1985). Abood and Milton's (1988) path-analytic model revealed that health practices/behavior and social support networks had statistically significant direct negative effects on illness. Dimensions of support (discussed in Chapter 1) may influence health behavior. Both perceived and received support contributed to pregnant women's adherence to health behavior, although these factors act differently in buffering stress and promoting positive health behavior (Aaronson, 1989).

It is conceivable that negative interactions with others might balance supportive functions yielding negligible benefit (Gottlieb & Selby, 1989). Support intended to be positive can have negative outcomes such as reinforcement of poor health behaviors or demeaning, debilitating assistance. For example, friends who drink may not be supportive of another's efforts to stop drinking.

Theories introduced in Chapter 1 also can be invoked to interpret impact of support on health behavior. Social comparison can exert influence at five stages of health and illness: behaviors that prevent or induce illness, decisions about the meaning of symptoms, decisions about the treatment of symptoms, responses to professional care, and recovery from illness (Sanders, 1982). Hanson, Herggeler, and Burghen (1987) discovered an interaction between stress and social competence for diabetes control. Social competence was associated with good control of diabetes only in the presence of high stress, whereas parental support was associated with adherence to regimen. Other studies have shown strong associations between adjustment to diabetes regimen and social competence (e.g., Kaplan & Toshima, 1990). Empirical associations between support and health-related outcomes may reflect reverse causation or influence of confounded factors such as social competence. Studies of the interplay between individual coping behaviors and the expression of support from others would yield insights about the influence of these factors on health behaviors and health status, providing a basis for designing interventions to optimize social support and health behavior.

Dimensions of health beliefs, social support, and self-efficacy were examined in a prospective trial of health promotion with 215 patients (Kelly, Zyzanski, & Alemagne, 1991): "Support of family and others did not enter significantly into either prediction of motivation or behavior, but did have some relationship to efficacy experience and to at-risk status" (p. 318). This may have been due to the way support was measured. Zimmerman and Connor (1989) found that the greatest influences on health behavior in descending order were family members, friends and coworkers (sources of support), supportiveness, encouragement of maintenance, and others' health change/modeling (support types). Influence of support on health behavior was explained in terms of social learning and self-efficacy theory. Muhlenkamp and Sayles (1986) linked social support to self-esteem and positive health practices. Likewise, Hubbard, Muhlenkamp, and Brown (1984) found correlations between social support and health practices. However, Yarcheski and Mahon's (1989) replication of the causal model in these two nursing studies indicated problems with varied samples and concluded that social support had no direct effect on positive health behavior among adults.

Epidemiological studies also have assessed the relationship between social networks and health habits of adults. For healthy men and women, the more extensive their social integration, the better their health practices (Berkman & Breslow, 1990). Intervention studies have shown effects of support and family involvement on smoking cessation, weight loss, blood pressure control, and dietary intake (Mermelstein, Lichtenstein, & MacIntyre, 1983; Morisky et al., 1983; Morisky, DeMuth, Field-Fass, Green, & Levy, 1985; Ockene, Benfari, Nuttall, Hurwitz, & Ockene, 1982; Sexton et al., in press; Zimmerman & Connor, 1989).

> Mary is trying to give up smoking. Her coworkers at her former job frequently took smoking breaks. This was an acceptable recreational outlet and an opportunity to socialize. During the initial period of separation Mary has increased her consumption of cigarettes from one-half to one pack a day. However, two factors

led to her desire to abstain: her recent bout with pneumonia and peer pressure encountered by her teenage daughter to start smoking herself. Mary's best friend and mother, both nonsmokers, are supportive of her efforts. Likewise, the support group members are valuable role models in that they have a nonsmoking rule for their meetings and social events.

Impact of Social Support on Health-Care Use

As noted in Chapter 1, social networks may affect help seeking and the use of health services through a variety of mechanisms. Utilization is a function of the relationship or complementarity between the organization of a professional service and the help-seeking pattern of laypersons (Birkel & Reppucci, 1983; Friedson, 1983). Informal networks can affirm the necessity to seek assistance through affirmational or appraisal support (Antonucci & Depner, 1982).

The social network may be viewed as part of the helping system; seeking lay support may be the initial step to seeking professional help (Wilcox & Birkel, 1983; Wills, 1983). Different network components provide different kinds of aid (Hammer, 1983; Litwak, 1985). Low users of health services may have dense networks of friends and kin (Garbarino, 1980; McKinlay, 1982). Weak ties are a chief impetus for entry to services (Auslander & Litwin, 1990; Gourash, 1978). Auslander and Litwin (1990) found that applicants for social services have significantly smaller networks and less affective support.

Cantor's (1979) Hierarchical Compensatory Model and Litwak's (1985) Task Specific Model explain factors that lead persons to prefer certain support providers and to seek help from others in an orderly fashion when the preferred providers are unavailable or unwilling (Rook, 1990). The propensity to seek help and to communicate needs influence receipt of support (Dunkel-Schetter & Wortman, 1985; Eckenrode, 1983; Heller & Swindle, 1983). Persons who wait for support to be offered may receive less support than they anticipated (Eckenrode, 1983). Positive beliefs about help seeking and internal locus of control are associated with greater support mobilization (Dunkel-Schetter & Bennett, 1990). Hobfoll and Freedy (1990) report how social support skills were increased by providing information on when and how support should be sought. People dealing with stressful life events tend to seek help first from their network of family and friends, before seeking help from professionals competent to deal with a particular problem (DePaulo, 1982). Some evidence indicates that support is least available when the stressors are most severe.

Problems in seeking support such as threat to self-esteem, learned helplessness, management of strong and weak ties, and relationship costs (Albrecht & Adelman, 1987) also may influence help seeking from professionals. Attribution and equity theories explain reactions to help seeking. Aid can be debilitating when the recipient has no opportunity to reciprocate, as is exemplified in professional relationships (DePaulo, 1982; Fisher et al., 1983). According to Lenrow and Burch (1981), social support is not conveyed in interactions between professional helpers and their clients because mutual aid is absent. However, feelings of indebtedness may be diminished, because professionals receive compensation. Other similarities and differences between professional and lay helpers influence use of health-care services.

Comparison of Formal and Informal Aid

Comparisons of professional and layperson aid suggest that the major differences can be categorized according to knowledge base, model of care, status/control, and ideology. Borkman (1976) distinguished professional knowledge from experiential knowledge as being theoretical and segmented rather than pragmatic and holistic. Seeing peers as role models is one element of experiential knowledge, which is developed within self-help groups through a process of individuals reflecting upon and trusting their firsthand experiences in the context of other people with similar experiences (Borkman, 1982, 1984). In contrast, a professional is viewed as a person committed to empirical and systematic knowledge (Lenrow & Cowden, 1980). Herein lies an essential difference between professionals and self-help group members.

Professional and lay helpers/groups both have articulated unique models of helping (Whittaker & Garbarino, 1983) and a desire to promote well-being (Katz, 1981; Maguire, 1983; Zarem, 1982). Professionals usually espouse values of society and promote incremental changes. In contrast, peer resources have differing values and may promote more radical changes (Fisher et al., 1988). Toro's (1986) comparative study of natural and professional help revealed similar helping strategies and effectiveness. Tracey and Toro (1989) later reported that the process of the helping interactions and the sequencing of behavior in response to the client, however, differed. Successful mutual-help leaders focused more on emotional support, self-disclosure, and questions following "experiencing" statements. In contrast, successful professionals used interpretations after description and not after experiential statements. Toseland, Rossiter, and Labrecque (1989) contrasted groups led by professionals and those led by peers. Both types facilitated caregivers' ability to deal with interpersonal concerns, improved their relations with the care receiver, decreased problems of caregiving, and increased their networks and knowledge of community resources. A 1-year follow-up of caregivers (Toseland, 1990) indicated that both types of groups were equally supportive. Toseland et al. (1989) report that both professional and peer-led support groups were effective at improving caregivers' coping ability and feelings of self-efficacy. Although professionals provided more help with coping skills and specific problems, no differences were evident in group outcomes.

A number of other empirical studies compare professionals and nonprofessionals along diverse dimensions (e.g., Bliwise & Lieberman, 1984; Brown, 1978; Cherniss & Cherniss, 1987; Durlak, 1979; Kurtz, 1984; Kurtz, Mann, & Chamber, 1987; Lieberman & Mullan, 1978; Manthei, 1982; Marmar, Horowitz, Weiss, Wilner, & Kaltreider, 1988; Ryan, 1985; Stuart & Mitchell, 1978; Thompson, Gallager, Neis, & Epstein, 1983; Toro, 1986; Toro et al., 1988; Yoak & Chesler, 1985), predominantly effectiveness in terms of outcomes and ideological differences. The reported similarities between the professional and nonprofessional groups are skills, attendance, atmosphere, outcomes (physical, emotional, knowledge, behavior), and rated effectiveness. According to these empirical studies, professionals and professionally led groups value objectivity, education, science, and traditional service models; have clientele/members who have experienced more stressful events; use open questions and reflections as helping-relationship skills; produce positive outcomes of increased satisfaction, knowledge, and social contact and decreased psychiatric symptoms; believe that the self-help modality is effective for only a few behavior-control problems; and remain in asymmetrical relationships with laypersons. In contrast, nonprofessional self-help group members value mutuality, shared problem solving and responsibility, and informal structure; use support, role modeling, self-disclosure, warmth, information, rapport, social monitoring, and outreach; consider that self-help can be useful for all problems; offer specific help; and focus on decreasing professional-member status and control distances.

Empirical comparisons of helping models and ideologies, types of knowledge bases, status, and control reveal differences and similarities. Nevertheless the functions of lay helpers and professionals appear to be complementary, consistent with balance theory premises. Health professionals, therefore, need to acknowledge and accommodate lay help movements and changes in health-care delivery that press for professional role change consistent with social support.

Significant Shifts in Society and Health-Care Delivery

Increase in Consumer Control and Self-Help Mutual-Aid Movements

Self-help and mutual aid have proliferated as part of the power-to-the-people movement (Rappaport, 1985) and the consumerism movement (Froland, 1980). The two major themes in the development of self-help groups are disillusionment with existing professional services and the decline of supportive institutions (Hatch & Kickbusch, 1983; Miller, 1983). The upsurge of self-help groups is related to disenchantment with professional experts and perception of depersonalization, overspecialization, dependence, stigmatization, fragmentation, rigidity, neglect, elitism, and ineffectiveness within formal professional sectors (Gartner & Riessman, 1984; Marques, 1983). Self-help groups aim to demystify professional expertise (Katz & Levin, 1980) by shifting power to consumers (Gartner & Riessman, 1984) and by altering traditional roles of laypeople and professionals (Hatch & Kickbusch, 1983).

It is not surprising, therefore, that many self-help groups maintain a strong antiprofessional or aprofessional stance. Yet other self-help groups have been voluntarily developed and maintained with the direct assistance of professionals. More commonly, both groups are ambivalent and experience tensions in their relationships with each other (Lenrow & Burch, 1981). Many of the tensions experienced between formal and informal helpers evolve from their basic differences, discussed in the previous section.

The social movement literature provides one framework for analyzing this pressure for health professional reform. Social movements involve collective action directed toward social change and conflict expression between groups fighting for control of resources (Cohen, 1985; Gundelach, 1984; Melucci, 1984, 1985; Touraine, 1985). New social movements value autonomy, identity, and opposition to manipulatory control and bureaucratization (Offe, 1985). These movements tend to involve consumer/citizen "battles" against the establishment. Consumer movements have stimulated an increased sense of rights and empowerment. The need for new forms of knowledge (Melucci, 1985; Touraine, 1985) and social learning (Cohen, 1985; Ede, 1985) guide social movements.

Several ideas in the social movement literature (in addition to acknowledgment of social learning) have relevance for social support and self-help groups. Interestingly, new movements are labelled networks of groups and individuals sharing a collective identity (Donati, 1984; Melucci, 1984, 1985). Offe (1984) concluded that self-help initiatives "could come to play an important role as long as they were recognized as socially normal and vital" (p. 237). As self-care practices to promote optimum health and functioning can be taught or reinforced within self-help groups, the two are distinct but related phenomena, and both are expressed in social movements. Clearly the self-help and self-care movements satisfy the following social movement criteria: decentralized units connected personally and structurally, an ideology, real or perceived opposition from society or the established order (Smith & Pillemer, 1983), a sense of common purpose, and action. Self-help groups in general are characterized by the need for both individual and social change (Katz, 1981; Katz & Bender, 1990). The self-help movement could be expected to affect the provider-consumer relationship and the preparation and education of health-care professionals.

Control of expert services by consumers is considered one alternative to professional and bureaucratic control (Derber, 1982; Reuschemeyer, 1983). In fact, Larson (1977) suggests that "lay clientele . . . could attack medicine's corporate power politically with the strength of a social movement" (p. 39). The issues raised by such movements are those connected with shifting boundaries (Cohen, 1985) between professional providers in the formal sector and lay helpers and consumers in the informal sector. As Katz (1985) predicted, "the self-help phenomenon is here to stay" and professionals must pay attention to how "mutual aid ideas and organizations . . . can be more fully used in serving clients" (p. 1).

Clearly, laypeople are increasingly unwilling to depend solely on professional expertise and ethics (McKinlay, 1982; Schon, 1983). An eminent social support researcher (Gottlieb, 1985b) identifies one reason: "Professionals reflexively and somewhat arrogantly presume that they have exclusive title to effective helping skills" (p. 20). This arrogance is based in part on the medical model.

Shift From Medical Model to Social Model

Nevertheless some health professionals continue to depend on the medical model (Clarke, 1986; Ryan, 1985). Health professionals were traditionally socialized in the expert care-provider role associated with the medical model. The traditional medical model has been criticized because of the inherent asymmetrical professional/patient relationship in which recipient dependence is fostered and professionals govern client behavior (Barbarin & Chesler, 1986; Crowenwett & Brickman, 1983). According to this model, people, as victims of disease, are not responsible for solving their own problems but must comply with experts treating their malfunctioning body parts (Brickman et al., 1982; Wright, 1979). In fact, most professional-treatment models depend on complex technologies (Lieberman & Bliwise, 1985) and a bioreductionist model that restricts comprehension of health problems to the function of the human organs (Laura, 1985).

Hence, many sectors of the health-care system continue to be preoccupied with cure and treatment rather than disease prevention and health promotion. Health-care budgets are devoted primarily to large- and small-scale hospitals and institutional settings and to care provided by medical practitioners. Community-based care has suffered from insufficient status and financial support (Canadian Nurses Association, 1988). Physical and mental health problems attributable to loneliness, social isolation, and alienation are increasing.

The World Health Organization (1984) lists "strengthening of social networks and social supports" as a health promotion strategy (Kickbusch, 1986). Augmenting the supportive resources available to all members of a community is congruent with the current aims of health promotion, described as involving self-care, mutual aid, and healthy environments (Epp, 1986). This reconceptualization of the health domain stresses health promotion, not illness cure. Further, the

World Health Organization (1985) recommends primary health-care alternatives to the dominance of the medical model. Therefore a recent change in focus from problemization to normalization reflects a shift from medical to social or health-focused models.

Move Toward Primary Health Care and Health Promotion

Clearly the evolving health needs and accompanying service delivery constraints in contemporary society cannot be addressed by professional resources alone. Accordingly, primary health care, which reflects a philosophy of citizen involvement, is espoused increasingly by professionals. Components of primary health care—self-care, mutual aid, public participation, creation of supportive environments, teamwork with lay helpers, and community-based care—are compatible with social support.

Many investigations, reported earlier in this chapter, have demonstrated the impact of social support on health status and health behaviors. Nurses have related support specifically to health promotion, one principle of primary health care (see Chapter 5). Major constructs of health promotion include not only nutrition, weight control, exercise, physical fitness, and stress management but also social support (Boyle, 1989; Cox, 1986; Pender, 1987). The availability of network support promotes the adoption of health-enhancing behaviors.

Access to health services and health status—another principle of primary health care—is particularly problematic for the poor (Stewart, 1990a). Singh and Pandey's (1990) study revealed that social support did not moderate the negative impact of poverty on coping. The poor and nonpoor differ widely in their perception of susceptibility to health conditions, severity of conditions, and effectiveness of health services (Rootman, 1989; Shah, 1987). These factors are derived from the health promotion model (Melnyk, 1988) to explain why an individual might engage in preventive health action. Those who seek medical or dental care or join self-help groups tend to be well-educated, white, middle-class women (DePaulo, 1982; McKinlay, 1982).

Citizen and community participation in the health-care system attempts to balance power with professionals (Warner, 1981). The "ideal" of citizen and community participation in health-care planning, delivery, and evaluation has been acknowledged in health promotion and primary health care premises. Health professionals could acknowledge that the impediments to consumer or public participation include the client's social isolation and vulnerability when confronting bureaucratic organizations, the potential monopolistic nature of health services, the stigmatization of some illnesses, and tokenism in health boards. Self-help group membership may foster feelings of individual and collective efficacy and empowerment. In sum, these factors influencing use of health services, including social movements and shifts in health-care models and delivery modes, have an impact on health professional roles.

When Mary developed pneumonia, she was initially reluctant to contact a physician. Her Christian Science background and the independent work ethic of her parents led her to believe that she should be able to manage by herself without calling upon a health professional. However, as her symptoms progressed in severity, her confidant urged her to seek medical care. In fact, she recommended a specific physician and several who should be avoided, based on her personal experience in the past. Mary acted on her advice, thereby using the formal health-care system for professional knowledge and skills regarding her physical health status, while continuing to rely on her natural network and newly created network for experiential knowledge and emotional support. Thus, the merits of both formal and informal aid during a particularly stressful period were reinforced. Mary's selection of a compatible health-care professional was based on premises of a social or primary health care model, rather than those of a medical model, concerning public participation and consumer control.

Health Professional Roles Relevant to Social Support

Professional roles may need to be redefined to enable help seeking and to enhance relevance to contemporary consumer needs. Self-help mutual-aid groups, as one example of social support, differ in their openness to professional involvement (Marques, 1983), as observed earlier. When professionals do participate, they are cast in an ancillary or secondary role; the structure and mode of operation is under the control of members, who may in turn draw upon professional guidance (Klass & Shinners, 1983; Levy, 1978, 1983; Shumaker & Brownell, 1984). Accordingly, virtually all reviews of linkages between formal and informal helping point to fundamental shifts and redefinitions in professional roles. These differ in significant ways from the direct-service roles played in traditional professional-client relationships.

Seven studies measuring self-help group members' perceptions and 12 studies of professionals' views, reviewed by Stewart (1990d), indicate that professional interaction with self-help groups is desirable. Professional lack of information concerning self-help groups and lack of preparation for appropriate roles and skills, however, are commonly perceived barriers. Relevant skills are community organization, group process, and consultation (Black & Drachman, 1985). The three professional roles vis-à-vis self-help groups most commonly identified by professionals were consultant, creator/catalyst, and referral resource (Stewart, 1990d). Two of these are not unexpected in light of admonitions to limit direct professional contribution; clearly consultation and referral are indirect functions. However, the frequent reference by professionals to the professional's directive role in initiating self-help groups is surprising, in view of the desire of most self-help groups for indirect professional involvement.

It is clear in studies of perceptions of group members (Gottlieb, 1982a; Levy, 1983; Marques, 1983) and those of professionals (Black & Drachman, 1985; Hermalin et al., 1979; Miller, 1983) that the indirect, nonauthoritarian, nondirective role of the professional as consultant receives the most support. Consultative assistance is offered only when it is desired and invited by membership (Jeger, Slotnick, & Schure, 1982). The consultee is free to use or not use the consultative help. Consultation necessitates a voluntary, coordinative relationship and is task oriented, regarding a circumscribed problem within a limited time span. Professional consultative and coordinating behaviors enhance collaboration by decreasing the social distance between professionals and self-help groups (Miller, 1983). Jacobs and Goodman (1989) predict that expanded professional consultation is an expected outgrowth of legitimization of the self-help mutual aid model and of its empowerment by the health-care system.

Empowerment is the endowment or enabling of clients and their network members with the authority and strength to effect decisions, behaviors, and interventions. It implies a sense of control, esteem, and collective efficacy for laypersons and lay helpers and can result from social movements and from reciprocal interchange with professionals. Empowerment is based on genuine collaboration among professionals and self-help group members, who are viewed by professionals as resources, not as clients (Rappaport, 1985). As Gottlieb (1982a) maintains, "ultimately their [self-help groups'] empowering effect stems from the sense of confidence and competence they instill, and from the dignity restored to people when they experience change at their own hands rather than at the hands of professionals." Health professionals should be teaching people how to achieve greater self-control and fulfillment through, for example, sharing professional and experiential knowledge.

Some may argue that there should be no roles for professionals from the formal sector vis-à-vis the informal sector. Feared risks to lay helpers and lay help groups include co-optation and domination by professionals, competition from professionals, appendage to a professional service, socialization in the professional mode, and conversion to poorly trained professionals (see, for example, Gartner & Riessman, 1984; Gottlieb, 1985a; Lieberman & Bliwise, 1985). There is "something inconsistent about a demystification of professional expertise which leads to the establishment of a breed of counter professional experts" (Schon, 1987, p. 342).

In short, the impetus and need for transformation of health professional roles is implied by social movements and shifts in models and delivery mechanisms. There appears to be general agreement in the literature that professionals should support and not supplant or coopt informal helping efforts, that methods should be sought for greater cooperation and communication between formal and informal health systems, and that professional education is a significant method (see Chapter 7). Moving from expert provider to equal partner will require basic modifications of roles and role preparation (Black & Weiss, 1990; Stewart, 1990c).

Summary

The impact of support on physical and psychological health status is indeed complex. Several models—main, moderating, and mediating—postulate pathways. The main effect is partially explained by the intricate relationship with the immune system. Deficient networks have a clearly demonstrated immune-suppressive effect. Types of relationships—intimate, nonreciprocal, or problematic—within the network influence health outcomes. However, poor health seems to have a bidirectional impact with the network by depleting resources.

Social networks affect health behavior through information, modeling, and encouragement. Social comparison, social competence, and social learning are germane mechanisms. Finally, social networks influence use of health services. Increase in "consumer control" social movements and shifts toward social and primary health care models are compatible with health professionals' accommodation of lay helpers. This adjustment necessitates a transition from traditional superior roles to more equitable linkages with the informal support networks of clientele.

❖ CHAPTER THREE ❖

Relevance of Social Support to Nurses
An Overview

Introduction

There are at least seven reasons that social support should be considered germane to the nursing profession. Nurses can acknowledge the potentially powerful impact of supportive resources on client maintenance of health, participation in care, and adaptation to chronic illness and recovery from acute illness; the ongoing interaction of individual clients with intimates and other social-network members; the accessibility of these network members to the nurse; and the influence of these informal helpers on use of nursing services and personal occupational stress. These premises could underlie theoretical frameworks that enrich nurses' understanding of the support phenomenon and could be operationalized in nursing empirical studies and intervention strategies. It would seem that nurses are in an excellent position to advance the study of social support.

Impact on Client Health and Health Behavior

In terms of sheer numbers, nurses are the largest source of health-care service in a delivery system that is becoming more oriented to health maintenance and promotion. Social support should be of particular interest to health professionals because of its impact on health behavior, on health status, and on health-services utilization. Berkman (1985) postulates that lay networks exert peer pressure on health behavior or lifestyle-related activities through individual choice. Considerable evidence shows that social support has direct (main) and indirect (buffering) effects on physical and mental health (Broadhead et al., 1983; Brownell & Shumaker, 1984; Cohen & Wills, 1985; Wallston, Alagna, & DeVellis, 1983). Clearly, social support is applicable to this evolving emphasis on healthy states.

The *buffering model* posits that support protects individuals from potentially harmful influences of acute stressful events and enhances coping abilities. Three pioneer authors of theoretical papers on social support (Caplan, 1976; Cassel, 1974; Cobb, 1976) supported the premise that available primary-group supports could "protect people in crisis from a wide variety of pathological states" (Cobb, 1976, p. 310).

The *main-effect model* proposes that social support directly benefits well-being by fulfilling basic social needs (Thoits, 1982) and social integration (Cohen & Wills, 1985). The main effect is equivalent to a primary preventive function and is explained in part by social inoculation theory. This theory posits that social support tends to make people less susceptible to some infections and neoplastic processes and that it does so by influencing some aspects of the humoral and cell-mediated immune response (Pilisuk, 1982). Conversely, disruptive life events can rend social networks and thereby suppress the immune system. The social support literature has only begun to consider the potential relationship of social support and immunity to disease and health. These indirect and direct effects of support on health outcomes were reviewed in Chapter 2.

Impact on Client Participation in Care

Another relevant trend in health-care delivery (discussed in Chapter 2) is consumer involvement, evidenced in the primary health care movement. Increasingly on international fronts self-care, mutual aid, strengthened social networks, and public participation are lauded as mechanisms for imparting primary health care and health promotion on a widespread basis (World Health Organization, 1978, 1984). The nursing profession has shifted to an espoused philosophy that clients should actively participate in their own care; social support in forms such as family, friends, indigenous lay helpers, neighbors, volunteers, and mutual-aid self-help groups is compatible with this premise. Social support premises reflect a lay helping philosophy. Effective public participation requires that nurses be knowledgeable about community and family interrelationships and willing to participate in a partnership relationship with communities to develop mechanisms to promote increased client self-care and self-reliance.

Blending professional practices with the cultural beliefs and practices of laypersons is germane to the implementation of primary health care (Baumgart, 1982). The professional relationship with clientele should be facilitative rather than prescriptive, and consultative rather than authoritarian. In a collaborative relationship, the agendas of client and nurse receive equal hearing. There is mutual goal setting and implementation of a negotiated plan of action.

Impact on Client Coping With Chronic Health Conditions

Third, the prevalence of chronic illnesses among nurses' clientele poses problems of social isolation and dependence with attendant familial and role-related stressors. Social support can alleviate the feelings of loneliness associated with disease and disability. Furthermore, unmet needs for support increase human vulnerability to physical and psychological illness and prolong recovery from illness (Bloom, 1990; Gottlieb, 1985a; Wortman & Conway, 1985). Nurses should find that social support is a valuable adjunct to their psychosocial-physiological knowledge of healthy states and of chronic and acute illness.

The review of nursing research on social support in Chapter 5 reveals that nurses have, to date, studied populations central to their profession's activities and concerns. They have contributed significant empirical studies of support resources and target populations, uniquely focusing on the acutely and chronically ill, as well as expectant couples, new parents, and the bereaved. Some at-risk groups have been more neglected, such as children, native peoples, the poor, the unemployed, and victims of abuse. Nurses practice in diverse institutional and community-based sites, and hence have direct contact with all these population groups. Broader theoretical frameworks, such as loneliness or social exchange, enhance understanding of the support process experienced by the chronically ill and their caregivers.

Environmental Support of Clientele

Fourth, nursing studies human wholeness or health because it recognizes that people and their environment interact continuously (Fawcett, 1989). Certainly the social environment of consumers of nursing services encompasses the support rendered by these consumers' social networks of friends, families, and others.

Most nursing models focus on a selected aspect of the environment (Ellis, 1982). The environment frequently is portrayed as a source of stressors, rather than a source of resources. Nursing care can encompass manipulation of the environment and environmental-person interactions (Ellis, 1982; Meleis, 1985). Furthermore, nursing actions are created, developed, modified, and constrained within given environmental contexts (Kim, 1983b). Therefore the environment, as the context of nursing practice and nursing's clientele, should be a focus of theoretical thinking in nursing.

However, the review in Chapter 6 demonstrates that nurse theorists have not clearly articulated or elaborated upon the concept of environment (Chinn & Jacobs, 1987; Chopoorian, 1986; Flaskerud & Halloran, 1980; Meleis, 1991) and have given the complex of structures and relationships that makes up the environment only peripheral attention and action (Chopoorian, 1986). Frequently, nursing deals with people who are experiencing, anticipating, or completing transitions that are situational, developmental, or health-illness events (Meleis, 1985). Nursing should not isolate the transition of an individual, a family, or a community from the environment.

Clearly, the concept of environment must become prominent in nursing theory. Chopoorian (1986) suggests reconceptualization of environment as human social relations. Theories centering on the environment could describe environmental properties, components, and dimensions that help maintain and promote health (Meleis, 1991). The time is ripe for explication and application of this critical concept, primarily in its social domain, because of its suitability to social support.

Accessibility of Nurses to Clients' Social Networks

A fifth factor is suggested in Gottlieb's (1985a) reference to "nursing's easy entrée to clinical settings and firsthand contact with patients and families." Caplan (1976), a pioneer in the social support field, also recognized nurses' frequent and intimate communication with clients and families. Nurses can use this accessibility of social-network members to enhance the supportive resources available to their clientele.

Nurses can validate concepts of social support in real-life situations with real-world populations. Nurses, through direct contact with clientele and their networks in health-care facilities and community-based sites, are particularly familiar with diverse populations. Thus they can realize the ideal of participant observation (Susskind & Klein, 1985). By having less intrusive entrée to community contexts, nurses can maintain face-to-face relationships with, and thus share the perspective of, the persons experiencing the problem. Applied/ intervention research conducted by nurses should enhance practical development of the social support field.

Support interventions are "efforts to optimize the psychosocial resources which individuals proffer and receive in the context of their relations with their primary social field" (Gottlieb, 1988a). Chapman and Pancoast (1985) distinguish interventions that increase network size, change the structure of the network, reinforce existing relationships, change the content of exchanges, or create ties between formal and informal systems. Regrettably, nurses rarely report facilitation of neighborhood helpers, volunteers, or community groups. A review and prospectus of nursing support interventions with natural and created networks, in practice and in research, appear in Chapters 4 and 5.

Impact of Client Network on Use of Nursing Services

Like other health professionals, nurses need to consider the impact of social networks on client utilization of and satisfaction with their services. The acceptable and relevant roles and intervention strategies with respect to these informal sources of support must be elucidated.

A World Health Organization (WHO) Study Group (World Health Organization & International Council of Nurses, 1987) recently classified components of the nursing role in primary health care as direct care provider, educator of the public, manager of services, and researcher or evaluator of health care. The extension of the natural role of nurses in primary health care should enable them to promote participation of individuals, families, and community groups in their own health development; to work more effectively with the community in coordinating health development with development in other sectors; to encourage the community to participate actively in developing and implementing health services; and to teach health concepts and self-care techniques. Thus professionals need to learn a partnership orientation to consumers and lay helpers. Indeed, consumerism and lay support movements (described in Chapter 2) will have a major impact on use of nursing services.

Impact of Social Support on Nursing Occupational Stress

Finally, the beneficial effects of social support on nurses experiencing occupational stress have been documented in intensive care settings (Norbeck, 1985c, 1985d; Oehler, Peter, & Sehler, 1989), nursing homes (Cohen-Mansfield, 1989), schools of nursing (Fong, 1990), and community health sites (Stewart, 1992). Perceived availability of support, emotional support, appraisal support, and duration of relationships were inversely related to nursing burnout (Cronin-Stubbs & Rooks, 1985; Firth, McIntee, McKeown, & Britton, 1986). Browner (1987) reports that the extent to which nursing staff could count on help from coworkers influenced their attitudes about their jobs, their coping, and their health.

Gottlieb (1982b) contends that occupational support from workmates protects workers from adverse health consequences of job stressors and influences coping with these stressors. Support from staff at work can be conceived as organizational or interpersonal (Firth et al., 1986). Evidence also shows that the support of coworkers significantly affects work satisfaction (LaRocco, House, & French, 1980). Job satisfaction is a continuing concern for nurses. (Chapters 4 and 5 examine the significance of occupational support to nurses and relevant research conducted by nurses.)

Significance of Social Support for Nursing Practice, Theory, Research, and Education: An Introduction

Nursing Practice

Most nursing services are offered in acute-care facilities and are focused on individuals rather than groups or communities. This reflects the service delivery system. It is conceivable that this problem also arises because nurses used to be "trained" in the medical model and institutional mode. Thus nurses may have been socialized in the expert role. Nurses, like other health professionals, may resist reallocation of power and removal of status differentials with respect to consumers of services and lay helpers.

The World Health Organization and the International Council of Nurses (1987) recently have recommended preparation of nurses for a new primary health care role, based on a premise of public participation. It is anticipated that nurses, therefore, will need to be socialized toward a new collaborative, partner role with consumers. Nurses can have significant collaborative roles with "created" networks such as self-help groups, as well as with "embedded" natural networks of family and friends.

From the professional viewpoint, the growing phenomenon of self-help groups is a social movement that challenges professional beliefs, methods, and expertise (Todres, 1982); shifts power to consumers (Gartner & Riessman, 1984); and alters traditional roles of laypeople and professionals. This points to the responsibility of nurses to acknowledge and accommodate consumer interests and to redefine their practice roles accordingly.

Conceptualization of the role of the nurse should emphasize a move toward consultant, partner, and primary health care roles, rather than "expert" institutionalized care of ill individuals. Norbeck (1981) suggests adapting the four steps of the nursing process (i.e., assessment, planning, intervention, and evaluation) to interaction with natural support networks. Nursing collaboration with lay helpers (e.g., volunteers, self-help groups, and family members) and consumers is also expedient. Furthermore, nurses can be involved in temporarily providing surrogate support in crises. However, the more usual nursing interventions in practice are to mobilize, to facilitate, and to enhance social networks. (See Chapter 4 for a more detailed discussion.)

The indirect consultant, partner, and facilitator roles at aggregate and community levels are emphasized in the social support literature. This orientation contrasts with the more direct service and expert nursing roles advocated in traditional nursing models. Collaborative rather than coexisting, co-opting, or conflicting modes of professional/social network interaction (Froland, Pancoast, Chapman, & Kimboko, 1981) are consistent with a social support model of practice. The view represented in many nursing models is more closely aligned with the coexisting mode.

Nursing Theory and Conceptual Models

Current conceptual models in nursing neglect the environmental domain, critical to any discussion of social support and mutual aid. No nursing theories concentrate on groups or the community, and few consider the family. The perspective of the consumer does not enter into nursing models. According to Hardy (1986), the consumer's (person's) world view has to be elicited because it may conflict with professional nursing views. These criticisms of existing theories, constructed by nurses, point to the need for a social support-based framework.

Nevertheless there is beginning recognition by nursing-theory analysts of the potential merits of social support theories and research. Meleis (1991) identifies Norbeck as an example of an author who viewed nursing via another paradigm: social support. Fawcett (1989) invoked the social support literature to exemplify descriptive, explanatory, and predictive theories. (See Chapter 6 for a more complete consideration of the significance of social support to nursing theory and of its potential for framing nursing science.)

There are clear commonalities and distinctions in conceptualizations of nursing support and social support. Both can have a health protective impact. Each can encompass the four major functions of social support identified by House (1981). Although both can include modelling and feedback, informational nursing support is based on technical and theoretical knowledge, whereas informational lay support includes experiential knowledge. Nursing support is a formal, professional source of support. Social support, although generally derived from informal, lay sources, occasionally and temporarily can be obtained from formal sources. Intimacy, social companionship, and social participation facets of social support (Barrera, 1986) are necessarily missing from nursing support. Further, nursing support lacks the reciprocal exchange of support resources between the individual and network members(s) deemed desirable in social support. However, mutual obligation, a characteristic of social support, is implied when nurses contract with clients.

Nursing Research

Nurse researchers (Brandt & Weinert, 1981; Cronenwett, 1985a, 1985b; Norbeck, 1985b, 1988a; Norbeck, Lindsey, & Carrieri, 1981, 1983; Tilden, 1985a, 1988; Weinert, 1987; Weinert & Brandt, 1987) have made significant strides in operationalizing the social support construct, contributions recognized by non-nurse experts (e.g., House & Kahn, 1985). The major components are encompassed within their measurement instruments. For example, Cronenwett (1985a) operationalized House's (1981) conceptualization of four types of support: emotional, appraisal, informational, and instrumental (material). Drawing upon Kahn and Antonucci (1980), Norbeck et al. (1981) operationalized three forms of social support: aid, affirmation, and affect (see Chapter 5.)

Thus nurses have illuminated the conceptualization of this important phenomenon through their research. For example, Hubbard et al. (1984) described the relationship between social support and self-care practices via a correlational study of senior citizens. Brown (1986b) empirically tested a conceptually derived formulation of social support with a sample of expectant couples. Multidimensionality of the construct was not confirmed. This finding is supported by nurse researchers (McNett, 1987; Norbeck, 1985b). In contrast, Barrera (1986), a psychologist, purports that the global concept of social support should be abandoned in favor of more precise concepts such as social embeddedness, perceived support, and enacted support.

Nurse researchers have contributed conceptual clarification, measurement devices, and empirical studies of support resources and target populations to the social support field. Nurse investigators contribute to the social support literature, primarily through research with clinical populations encountered in nursing practice (Norbeck, 1988b). Some nursing studies have examined occupational support for nurses working in a variety of sites and roles.

Most nursing studies have simply examined the social support currently existing in the natural environment that the respondent has actually received or perceives as a potential resource. However, nurses in empirical studies in the extensive literature reviewed had, with seven notable exceptions, not intervened to facilitate, enhance, or mobilize the informal networks of the target populations. Furthermore, only two used a true randomized control trial design. (Target populations, measuring instruments, and correlational intervention studies by nurses are detailed in Chapter 5.)

Nursing Education

Finally, nurse educators may be beginning to respond to the challenge of integrating social support theory into educational curricula. Tilden (1985b) descriptively analyzed the social support content incorporated into the curricula of the undergraduate and graduate programs of one university school of nursing in the United States, but cautioned that the findings only suggested trends and could not be considered either representative or conclusive. King (1984) and Santora (1983), who contrasted conceptual frameworks of baccalaureate with other nursing programs, found that the use of environmental terms such as *social system* was inconsistent. The environmental domain, as noted earlier, also has been neglected in practice models.

A study of the learning needs of a sector of the Canadian nursing population regarding lay support groups recently was conducted. The reported deficits in nurses' knowledge of specific mutual-aid groups and characteristics and benefits of the self-help modality, in requisite community organization and consultation skills, and in relevant role assumption point to the need for undergraduate and continuing education (Stewart, 1989a). A concurrent examination of the relevant curriculum foci of Canadian university schools of nursing (Stewart, 1988) indicated that there could be increased emphasis on the natural tensions between professionals and nonprofessionals and on partnership relationships.

Interdependence of professionals with clients, and sensitivity to the views of clients, should become principles of professional education (Lenrow & Burch, 1981). However, Katz (1985, p. 134) recommends that professional curricula emphasize self-help forms until this vision of interdependence is realized.

A brief commentary on pertinent classroom and clinical student learning opportunities and teaching strategies appears warranted. In the classroom and tutorial context, selected content foci that could be relayed didactically include the relevance of social support to health professionals and nurses, major theoretical viewpoints concerning social support, theoretical and empirical contributions of nurses to the social support literature, and appropriate roles of professionals. In tutorial sessions, students can be guided to examine their own experiences with informal helping (Gottlieb & Farquhason, 1985). Group experiences in tutorials or seminars should help nursing students to develop skills for use with self-help groups. Experiential learning opportunities, through field assignments/clinical placements, should also prepare student nurses for assuming appropriate primary health care roles. Role modeling by faculty and by student role playing can facilitate this experiential process.

Farquharson (1987) legitimately laments that professionals are socialized and educated as though professional knowledge were all that can be known about the domain of professional practice, when in fact experiential knowledge drawn from personal experiences is an important ingredient. At the same time, he asserts, professionals constantly must share their professional knowledge base as much as possible because doing so will empower others toward greater self-control and fulfillment. Clearly students should learn to empower clients and their social networks. (The educational implications of social support for nursing are explicated in Chapter 7.)

Summary

Thus the stage is set in the theoretical, research, practice, and educational spheres of the nursing profession for a framework derived from social support premises. As Tilden (1985c) claims, social support is socially congruent because people increasingly want to have greater involvement, authority, and responsibility for their own health care, and because society desires more humane and personalized health care that keeps natural networks intact during times of illness, crisis, and transition. The expectations of society and of consumers, citizens and lay helping networks, in all probability could be fulfilled through nurses developing, testing, and applying a social support framework.

❖ CHAPTER FOUR ❖

Nursing Practice
Significance of Social Support

Social support is relevant to nursing practice in hospital and community sites. Nurses play important roles in enhancing and mobilizing their clients' support. In doing so, they assess support needs, plan interventions, intervene at a variety of levels, and evaluate the effects of these interventions. Furthermore, nurses themselves need support to ameliorate the stress of practice in a variety of sites and roles.

Relevant Roles of Nurses

Nurses indirectly mobilize and enhance support provided by focal networks and directly provide supplementary, "surrogate" support—replacing inadequate or unavailable support in the network (Norbeck, 1988a)—during periods of stress, crisis, or transition (Stewart, 1989e). Nurses play consultant (facilitator), liaison, educator, and advocate (empowerment) roles, in addition to traditional care-provider roles (see Chapter 6 for definitions of roles). The consultant role encompasses educational, counseling, and facilitative functions. Nurses frequently are described as facilitators of support groups

AUTHOR'S NOTE: The discussion of intervention strategies at varied levels builds on a 1989 article by the author published in *International Journal of Nursing Research.*

in both the hospital (e.g., Halm, 1990) and the community (e.g., Sanfilippo, Galbraith, & Yussman, 1989). They are also educators of consumers and their social networks. Counseling techniques are used by nurses in group therapy (e.g., Anderson, 1989; Pasquarello, 1990). The liaison or coordinator role helps to maintain continuity among clients and their professional and lay helpers and to coordinate practical aspects of support groups. Nurses can also refer to support groups (e.g., Selenkow, 1990). Finally, nurses can create groups or revitalize existing groups (Heiney & Wells, 1989).

Nurses' roles in support or self-help groups can be guided by social-psychological research. Professionals in support groups typically provide professional sanction and structure; offer expert information about the stressor, coping strategies and resources, and group dynamics; and mobilize resources of different community agencies (Gottlieb, 1988a). Professionals consider referral, initiator, trainer, speaker, support provider, and linking-agent roles appropriate. However, surveys of member opinions reveal a much lower acceptance of the initiator and networker/linker roles than do studies of professional perceptions. Consensus exists on the acceptability of the consultant and referral roles (Stewart, 1990d).

Nurses have indirect support roles not only with groups but also with individual clients and their families. Nurses can identify members of the social network whom clients can approach for help (Rheume & Gooding, 1991). They can focus clients' attention on finding new ways of reciprocating to prevent erosion of the network and increase self-esteem; help clients recognize their support needs and potential sources of support; facilitate positive interaction with others through suggestions and role modeling; directly mobilize social networks by undertaking contact or inviting network members to a planning conference; plan respite for family members; help family members evaluate whether their goals are attainable; and facilitate honest communication to reduce misunderstandings and stress in the network (Halm, 1990; Weinert & Tilden, 1990).

Nurses play more direct support roles, reflected in surrogate support and supportive behaviors. Nurses in the Barnard, Snyder, and Spietz (1984) study provided surrogate support for 60 new mothers who had multiple problems and needed support additional to that available from their network. Numerous supportive behaviors are identified in the literature reflecting the nurse's direct supportive role. Listening, information exchange, validation, valuing, connecting, empowering, preserving integrity, empathizing, suggesting tangible resources, availability, promoting comfort, giving information, and helping to solve problems (Davies & Oberle, 1990; Gardner & Wheeler, 1987; Garvin & Kennedy, 1990; Kirgis, Godfrey, & McNell, 1991; Sexton & Stephen, 1991) are diverse dimensions of the nurse's direct supportive role.

Gottlieb (1988a) declares that professionals "are teaching the skills required to initiate and maintain supportive peer relationships, animating the formation of support groups and partnerships, and augmenting the supportive provisions rendered by the social orbits in which people participate" (p. 23). This statement captures succinctly nursing practice roles, both indirect and direct, with respect to social support.

Nursing Process Applied to Social Support Roles

As the nursing process is the core of nursing practice, the applicability of social support to the four stages of this decision-making model (assessment, planning, intervention, and evaluation) is delineated next.

Assessment Phase

Nurses can learn to assess the complexity of enacted or perceived social support from the perspectives of social network members and clients and to assess its impact on health. Requirements for and satisfaction with support fluctuate over the life course (Schulz & Rau, 1985) in relation to different stressors and different stages of coping (Jacobson, 1986). Supports may be drawn from different sources for different problems (Gottlieb, 1987; Pearlin, 1985). Assessment, therefore, should focus on target populations, types of support available for different stressors, sources of support, timing and duration of support, costs and/or benefits associated with support, satisfaction with support, behaviors perceived as supportive, and the overall level of social support (also see Chapter 5). Attribution, social comparison, coping, equity, psychoneuroimmunology, and social learning theories (see Chapter 1) can be invoked in this assessment phase to analyze support gaps and deficiencies.

Nurses have used objective and subjective measures for assessing support (Ryan & Austin, 1989). Norbeck (1988a) points to the need to develop and validate brief social support measures for clinical assessment of at-risk individuals. Brandt (1984b) compares the Norbeck Social Support Questionnaire (NSSQ) and the Personal Resources Questionnaire (see Chapter 5) as assessment tools. Brandt suggests that network size, diversity, and stability; the content or type of help; and costs and benefits of activating social resources are particularly important for clinical assessment purposes. McGough (1990) and Dean (1989) adapted the NSSQ to assess support types and sources of different population groups. Barrera's Index of Socially Supportive Behaviors has been used to describe how often types of support were received (Dean, 1989). In addition to assessing network strength, availability of social relationships, and timing of support, the nurse should examine each client's personal characteristics (e.g., locus of control, attachment vs. social isolation, and personal strength) and socio-demographic characteristics to interpret relevant factors (Alley & Foster, 1990).

Assessment can be based on the empirical literature as well as preliminary cross-sectional community or target population surveys to provide empirical evidence of support needs (Sandler, Gersten, Reynolds, Kallgren, & Ramirez, 1988). Assessment may "reveal the existence of social ties that can be further developed along the helping dimension, as well as relationships that are conflictual and amplify stress" (Gottlieb, 1987, p. 24). Fisher et al. (1988) recommend assessment of underuse and overuse of support resources. Finally, assessment involves weighing the need for social support versus the actual social support available to determine whether the level of social support is adequate (Norbeck, 1981), thus providing a basis for planning.

> The community health nurse (CHN) working in Mary's district was notified when Mary was released from the hospital following a crisis pertaining to pneumonia. Preliminary assessment by the clinical nurse specialist in the hospital identified her apparently diminished and potentially strained network as a risk. The CHN had Mary complete Norbeck's instrument during her first home visit to assess the size and durability of Mary's social network and her evaluation of individual members' ability to proffer pertinent aid, affect, and affirmation. At the same time, Mary's social isolation and social skills were assessed. Finally, the

visiting nurse noted the strain and conflict in Mary's relationship with her ex-husband, the overuse of support from her mother, the burden of her role as mother of two needy children, and the diminished contact with former coworkers and some friends. Level of support therefore was assessed as inadequate, because available support was exceeded by imminent needs for support.

Planning Phase

Planning interventions typically begins with diagnosing the problem or support needs. Diagnosis will be based on assessment of the stressor (e.g., illness) within the context of the surrounding social network and of the client's ability to receive and provide support. The diagnosed problem might be social isolation, alterations in family processes, dysfunctional social interaction, powerlessness, diminished self-esteem, or ineffective coping (Alley & Foster, 1990; McGough, 1990; Tilden & Weinert, 1987). Thus the supportive requirements or deficiencies associated with the stressor (Gottlieb, 1988a) will be identified.

Norbeck (1981) maintains that when social support is determined to be inadequate, planning and intervention are done to influence the probable outcome; if social support is judged to be sufficient, no intervention is required. She identifies factors determining possible interventions as the network's capacity to change and the individual's requisite skills and attitudes.

Sandler, Gersten, Reynolds, Kallgren, and Ramirez (1988) depict how client input into the planning of support interventions was solicited systematically from bereaved children and their families. Participants were asked to comment on the helpfulness and desirability of 11 potential support-program elements (e.g., discussion groups, meeting someone in the same situation, suggested coping strategies, support person visiting or phoning, reviewing information, or practical advice). Hence, planning should entail the collaborative efforts of nurses, clients, and clients' social-network members to negotiate goals and respective roles and to make decisions about preferred intervention strategies.

Assessment by the clinical nurse specialist and the community health nurse yield a diagnosis of increased social isolation and diminished self-esteem for Mary and dysfunctional social inter-

> action for her children. In both cases, support interventions were deemed necessary. Hence the CHN suggests a support group of mothers who are recently separated or divorced in that community, after reviewing alternative interventions with Mary. A similar strategy is employed for planning support interventions for the two children.

Intervention Phase

Support interventions are defined by Gottlieb (1987) as "efforts to optimize the psychosocial resources which individuals proffer and receive in the context of their relations with their primary social field" (p. 4). Interventions can be designed to extend or enhance functioning of natural support networks (Norbeck, 1988a). Chapman and Pancoast (1985) distinguish interventions that increase network size, change the structure of the network, reinforce existing relationships, change the content of exchanges, or create ties between formal and informal systems. Professionals can facilitate personal networks, mutual-aid groups, neighborhood helpers, volunteer linkage, and community empowerment (Froland et al., 1981). It is noteworthy that the final three intervention strategies typically have been overlooked in the nursing literature.

More specifically, support interventions can (a) improve use of existing support resources by targeting negative attitudes and beliefs regarding help seeking, (b) develop and maintain support resources that best serve at-risk groups, (c) help families identify strengths and weaknesses, (d) contain costs by trimming networks of unreliable support, (e) establish new relationships, (f) maintain old relationships, (g) manage negative support incidents by intensive individual or group programs, and (h) enhance support appraisal for those prone to devalue ties (Vaux, 1990). To moderate the costs of seeking support when there is underuse of resources, opportunity for reciprocity or normalizing (when the problem is shared by others) can be proffered by professionals. Incremental success opportunities that enhance self-efficacy and perceived control can intervene when there is overuse of support resources (Fisher et al., 1988). Professionals can help family members validate the experience of affected persons and thus enhance the client's self-esteem and motivation regarding positive health behaviors (Coyne et al., 1988).

Interventions should be matched to assessed need. A needs-fit model of support effects proposes that received support should match the stressful situation to be beneficial (Cohen & Wills, 1985; Okun, Melichar, & Hill, 1990). Hence the goal of indirect support interventions can focus on reducing uncertainty and despondency, enhancing self-help and enabling skills, promoting adaptive coping, reducing hopelessness, restoring hope, exploring alternative solutions, and expanding the client's repertoire of coping behaviors. In designing interventions, consideration should be given not only to the stressor, but also to the desired intensity of the intervention, the client's other personal resources, the timing of the interventions in the stressor sequence, the type of support needed, the potential drain of resources in support networks, and the appropriate level of the intervention.

Levels of Intervention

Nurse authors have paid minimal attention to individual, dyadic, and group-level interventions and have overlooked social-system and community-level interventions completely. These terms, derived from Gottlieb's (1988b) typology of intervention levels, are used here as a guide to proposing social support intervention strategies for practice (which also could become the focus of future empirical study by nurses). These strategies encompass both nurses' indirect role in facilitating social support by strengthening or maintaining an existing social network or by grafting on new ties and their direct role in surrogate support.

Individual Level. Individual-level interventions focus on modifying how the individual elicits or evaluates support provided by others (Rook & Dooley, 1985) and on developing social skills necessary to form and sustain supportive peer ties. These interventions concentrate on modifiable dispositional factors constraining and enabling the expression of support, which may alert individuals to adopt coping strategies that are less socially alienating and more inviting of support from the network (Gottlieb, 1988a). The educational role of the professional is paramount. The focus is on help-seeking behaviors and attitudes. Such interventions have been used to help children develop prosocial skills (Gottlieb, 1988b), to train recently separated or divorced adults (Rook & Dooley, 1985), and to improve solitary skills that enhance coping with loneliness, as well as to facilitate social bonding through individual-centered therapeutic strategies (Rook, 1984). In the words of the old adage, "People may be lonely because they build walls instead of bridges."

> *Example: Support Recipient Skills.* The physical and mentally handicapped children in schools and those who are from low-income groups, abusive family situations, foster homes, single-parent homes, remote rural areas, and minority cultures (e.g., if there are only a few Native Americans in the school) can be identified by the nurse in schools as populations potentially at high risk for social isolation and loneliness problems. Client perceptions would need to be elicited to confirm or deny this tentative targeting. Individual-level interventions, with the nurse directly providing emotional, informational, and instrumental social support, could be initiated on a trial basis. In addition, the nurse could institute interventions that facilitate social bonding, social skills, and problem-solving skills through training to overcome loneliness.
>
> Pre- and post-treatment interviews could ascertain situational versus dispositional attributions regarding cause and solution of loneliness, degree of perceived loneliness and social isolation, and adaptation to the school environment. (Later, a buddy system could evolve, or groups of children with similar concerns could be established as alternative treatments.)

Dyadic Level. Dyadic, or "micro-level," support strategies can emphasize introduction of supportive lay companions who are strangers or confidants, or improvement of the amount, regulation, and quality of communication among professional caregivers, clientele, and the client's proximal network members. These interventions involve augmenting or intensifying particular kinds of support from a key network member, or matching and introducing an outsider to a recipient to facilitate a supportive alliance through a grafted tie. The most common examples are hospital-based volunteer visitor programs for myocardial infarction, mastectomy, and stroke victims; "labor coaches"; and community-based "compliance" and widow- to-widow programs (Gottlieb, 1985a, 1985c). People with similar problems and interests can be linked, and citizen volunteers and companions can be mobilized (Froland et al., 1981). These strategies facilitate emotional and instrumental support, in particular.

Example: Dyadic Mobilization of Support From Key Network Members. Dyadic interventions can be focused on the hospitalized child. Nurses in pediatric wards can regulate visiting hours and non-threatening private sites for visits by key members of the social network, including friends in the neighborhood and schoolmates, in addition to parents, siblings, and grandparents. They can all participate (with assistance) in physical care and provide emotional support. (These key caretakers could be offered respite.) Intentional linkage to the Sunday school teacher, members of the Sunday school class, and the schoolteacher might increase a sense of mastery of role-related functions. Initially, a modified version of Bryant's Neighborhood Walk assessment tool (Bryant, 1985) could be used to examine actual and potential sources of intimate, confidant support from different generations (peer, parent, grandparent). This could be supplemented by identifying social-network members who are sources of conflict more than support, those who have not been utilized in the past, and those not available but desired. Pairs of children with the same condition and approximately the same age could be linked (for example, as roommates), to facilitate sharing of problems and coping solutions; prosocial emphatic communication; situational attribution; and reciprocal emotional, appraisal, and instrumental aid. They could help each other in small caregiving tasks and homework. Expressed appreciation of services rendered also would be significant in this buddy system. These buddies could continue to retain contact after one is discharged and, after both are discharged, could communicate with the assistance of the liaison nurse or nurses working in the community.

Pre- and post-treatment evaluation of perceived and actual support, and of changes in positive and negative support, in social network size, and in duration of support, would be necessary. Follow-up in-depth, semistructured interviews at intervals would help the assessment of adaptational and emotional outcomes. In addition, observation of quality and frequency of interactions is possible in the hospital.

Example: Introduction of New Supportive Ties. A time-limited support intervention linked an individual who had successfully recovered from an aorta-coronary bypass graft (ACBG) with one about to undergo similar surgery. These individuals answered questions, provided specific information, and offered emotional support by listening and responding to concerns. Nurses served primarily as mobilizers and facilitators of the educative and supportive public relations, planning, and community-outreach activities assumed by the lay participants. An initial recruiting, screening, and orientation program was conducted by nurses (Meagher, Gregor, & Stewart, 1987). Most visits took place with the patient only, yet over time there was an increasing number of visits with the family present and with the family during the surgical period. The volunteers most commonly gave emotional, informational, and appraisal support.

Although the intervention was not conducted as a randomized trial, individuals hospitalized for ACBG surgery could be randomly assigned to an experimental or control group. The treatment group would be visited one day before surgery by someone who had fully recovered from the same surgery. A control group would be visited by nonspecific volunteers, to distinguish the effect of post-ACBG volunteers from any volunteer involvement. The subjects could be contacted during a home visit 2 weeks following discharge by their "hospital visitor" as a form of follow-up. Attitudes to lifestyle, activity status, and compliance pre- and post-program could be identified and contrasted. (Subsequently, a self-help group could be established by the lay visitors for ex-patients and their spouses.)

Group Level. Group, or "mezzo-level," interventions either optimize support rendered by the existing network or graft on a set of new ties for target populations at risk due to social isolation or losses from the social network. These interventions are dedicated to creating more robust and durable support systems for one or more of their members (Gottlieb, 1988b). Thus the existing informal network can be enlarged, restructured, intensified, optimized, and reinforced (Froland et al., 1981; Young, Giles, & Plantz, 1982) through training, linking/coordinating, and outreach efforts of professionals. One aim is to improve natural helpers' helping skills and hence promote local helping.

Programs that train laypeople to train other natural helpers in basic helping, empathic, and crisis-intervention skills (e.g., D'Augelli & Ehrlick, 1982; Froland et al., 1981; Young et al., 1982) have produced mixed results. The failure of training to generalize to naturalistic settings, described by D'Augelli and Ehrlick (1982), may occur because such programs usually are based on professional value systems, which may not be culturally congruent with target populations and may supplant and deplete natural network resources (Gottlieb, 1988b). Such pyramid models are cost-effective, efficient, and easy to evaluate, but introduce artificiality and social distancing (Rook & Dooley, 1985). Finally, social-skills training occasionally can occur in group format.

Another facet of group-level intervention involves optimizing the support rendered by the existing network. Network-centered interventions attempt to change features of the network without increasing the network size. The few such interventions that have been studied have been aimed at chronically stressful situations and involve network coaching, network sessions, and network construction (Gottlieb, 1988b). For example, families can be helped to understand the importance of the support provider being involved in activities and maintaining a support network outside the caregiver/care receiver relationship (Coyne et al., 1988). As potential conflicts may exist between the natural network and outside peer resources, professionals could suggest use of outside resources in conjunction with other sources of support (Fisher et al., 1988).

Example: Instrumental Support. Instrumental support could be offered to the low-income caretakers of the elderly through day-care centers, homemaker services, visiting nurses, training of neighbors or volunteers in the area, and other respite services facilitated by nurses in community health positions. Caretaker burnout, fatigue, guilt, and loss of freedom can be prevented by diffusing responsibility to churches, senior-citizen centers, and self-help groups in the area and by using respite-care centers and services. Linkage to one or more elderly persons in the neighborhood would promote emotional and informational support, and enhance coping skills. The aim would be to foster mastery and self-esteem. Furthermore, involvement of the elderly in foster grandparents programs would allow them to help a third party, which can be as beneficial as direct reciprocity. Appraisal support through social comparison in such programs would be an important by-product.

Grafting on a New Set of Ties

Support-group interventions, like network interventions, focus on constructing ties to optimize support but do this by adding new ties that are complementary or supplementary (Gottlieb, 1988b). The support offered is more specialized than the general support provided by family and friends. The support group is a professionally supported unit, formed and supervised by professionals, and open to specifically selected populations. Although they share features of self-help groups, support groups differ in that they have the presence of one or more professionals who blend expert information about the illness and its management with group-facilitation activity. Furthermore, they are usually time-limited, convened in institutional settings, and emphasize coping exclusively, rather than a blend of coping and advocacy (Gottlieb, 1985c). "The professional supplements the participants' experiential knowledge with expertise about the group process, the stressors members face, and the coping strategies that may be germane" (Gottlieb, 1988a).

> *Example:* Children with cystic fibrosis or chronic obstructive pulmonary disease could be randomly allocated to either a control group or a nurse-led support group offering professional and peer informational, appraisal, and emotional social support on a weekly basis. This could occur initially in pediatric hospital settings, with follow-up groups established in the community for those who have been discharged. Social comparison regarding coping strategies, role modeling, situational attribution, and mutual reciprocal aid would be emphasized, as well as comprehension of and conformance with health-care recommendations.
>
> Observations and interviews would occur periodically (e.g., biweekly). Follow-up monitoring of duration and frequency of extra-group contact and of long-term impact on adherence with complex regimen restrictions could be measured again by interview.

Anecdotal reports and descriptive studies of support groups suggest the range of target populations of group interventions. Nurses have led groups for cancer victims (Diekmann, 1988), for stroke survivors and their families (Pasquarello, 1990; Pierce & Salter, 1988), for infertile women (Sanfilippo, Galbraith, & Yussman, 1989), for relatives of mentally ill adults (Platt, 1990), for parents of young children (McConville, 1989), for parents of chronically ill children (Betz, Unger, Frager, Test, & Smith, 1990), for patients who are recipients of automatic implantable cardioverter defibrillators and their families (Teplitz, Egenes, & Brask, 1990), for inpatients with chronic mental illness (Kelly, Sautter, Tugrel, & Weaver, 1990), and for women suffering prenatal bereavement (Wheeler & Limbo, 1990). These groups all focused on information exchange, shared feelings, and emotional support. Regrettably, although observations of improvements were noted, no measures of effectiveness or outcomes were included in these reports. A few studies discussed tentative outcomes. Braden (1990) reported that self-help class attendance contributed to self-help behavior of persons with arthritis. Groups for persons with HIV/AIDS appear to enhance empowerment and decrease isolation and stigma (Ribble, 1989), consistent with Taylor, Falke, Mazel, and Hilsberg's (1988) observation of normalizing and social comparison and Powell's (1988) empowerment model. Finally, high levels of perceived support and more problem-focused than emotion-focused coping strategies were revealed in members of self-help ostomy groups (Rheume & Gooding, 1991).

Social System. According to Gottlieb (1988b), social system, or "macro-level," interventions consist of "role definitions entailing more continuous support . . . [and] organizational policy/structural changes aiding or removing barriers to expression of support." Restructuring of school settings for the lonely (Rook, 1984); providing community forums that have input into local policies; establishing local task forces that assess, plan for, and meet community needs; and coordinating local opinion and neighborhood leaders (Froland et al., 1981) represent examples of this level of intervention. Furthermore, complementary linkages between informal and formal networks can be created (Chapman & Pancoast, 1985).

Problems underlying health (e.g., poverty) can be addressed only by interventions at this level. Regrettably, nurses and other health professionals traditionally have avoided the policy arena. Yet "to ignore the broader context within which social ties operate . . . constitutes a political misuse of findings on social support and health relationships" (Pilisuk & Minkler, 1985). In fact, social-system interventions, due to their potential ecological and preventive impacts through the creation of more responsive and durable personal communities, may yield longer-term benefits than individual interventions (Gottlieb, 1988a).

Example: Role Definition. The role of the occupational health nurse could be expanded to encompass a social support function that could encourage identifying the lonely and socially isolated. Initially, occupational health nurses would assess whether the deficit is at the dyad or the social-network level. If a confidant is required, linkages of those with similar interests can be initiated. If a social network approach is needed, groups of those with specific health concerns, such as substance abuse (with its obvious employment implications), could be established. Further, encouragement of hiring of the handicapped and creation of pertinent support sources, and follow-up of the recently unemployed (those fired, on leave of absence due to illness, etc.) through peer and family contact, would be part of the role. Finally, educational sessions could focus on promotion of environmental changes that might facilitate communication between coworkers and administrators. The occupational health nurse would need to collaborate not only with work supervisors but also with employees.

The expanded role could be tested on a trial basis. Employees, families, and supervisors could be interviewed pre- and post-program regarding changes in social-network size and composition, types of positive support provided/used, and conflicted or negative support.

Example: Organizational/Structural Changes. Nurses can facilitate citizen participation in health-care delivery through boards of multiservice centers and volunteerism, can advocate facilities and resources for self-help and support groups, and can promote active grassroots involvement at the regional, local, and personal levels. Furthermore, health-care facilities can be modified to involve the family and friends of clientele. The empowerment dimension of self-help groups can be encouraged as a form of community development. For example, nurses can facilitate groups of individuals with conditions such as total allergy syndrome in contacting the media and in pressuring public health officials for third-party payment of treatment. The social isolation accompanying such illnesses could be overcome by lobbying for environmental manipulation of public places—such as smoke-free shopping malls, restaurants, and transportation systems. Environmental settings and organizations can be altered to promote interaction with others and accessibility to social support resources.

Community Level. Gottlieb (1988b) defines "macro-level" interventions as educational strategies promoting a network orientation to coping. Rook and Dooley (1985) describe this approach as "community utilization" and refer to mass education campaigns designed to create a climate favorable to help seeking and help giving among the public and to promote awareness and acceptance of social support. Hersey, Klibanoff, Lam, and Taylor (1984) report how articles, films, pamphlets, and media coverage can be used to promote social support and social-network frequency of interaction on a large scale. Community awareness and educational programs can help prevent loneliness by removing obstacles to social contact (Rook, 1984). Community-level interventions, like individual-level interventions, exclusively focus on informational support, and entail a high degree of professional involvement. The strategy is difficult to implement and evaluate because of lack of control of extraneous variables and problems in measuring process and outcome, difficulties prevalent in other primary-prevention and health-promotion programs.

Example: Educational Strategies. Professional nursing associations and individual nursing practitioners can use television to relay messages regarding the impact of social networks and social support on health and specific examples of such help. In addition, nurses can write articles in consumer magazines and newspapers, can describe the relevance of specific forms and sources of social support, and can encourage linkages in the community. For example, nurses could develop more health-relevant social-support messages akin to public service announcements promoting the importance of family life by religious groups. However, they could expand the natural network described to include other sources of social support, such as friends, neighbors, and coworkers. Furthermore, nurses can facilitate the outreach strategies and mass media educational services provided by voluntary self-help organizations, such as the Alzheimer's Society.

The media can be used to publicize the social support projects identified under the other four levels of intervention. The media can serve as a public forum for individuals and groups (lay and professional) to express their views and provide feedback on social support needs and resources. Further, community-level intervention should target populations at risk of deficient social support.

Outcome measures could include pre- and post-treatment surveys of percentages of people who belong to primary face-to-face groups, who engage in volunteer activities, or who participate in community social activities, clubs, and/or organizations that can promote cohesion and affiliation among citizens.

Multilevel Interventions. A multilevel intervention approach can reflect Rook and Dooley's (1985) underlying premise of multiple causation for complex social and health problems. Heiney, Ruffin, Ettinger, and Ettinger's (1988) multimodal nursing intervention for adolescents and their parents included group meetings, educational programs, and retreats for professionals and volunteers.

Example: A widower-to-widower support program, similar to Vachon, Lyal, Rogers, Freeman-Letofski, and Freeman's (1980) widow-to-widow program, could be established by nurses. This would sequence dyad and group-level support and later would add a social-system dimension. The system-level intervention would focus on advocacy for change regarding retirement income, housing, and recreational and transportation services, which in turn would enable the elderly to remain in the community. Linked professional and nonprofessional support services would help avoid relocation to an institution and the associated stress of such a move.

Long-term follow-up and evaluation interviews could focus on physical and psychological well-being outcomes. The latter could include loneliness and coping scales.

* * *

The CHN referred Mary to an established support group of mothers who met weekly to discuss problems associated with single parenthood and the associated need to seek employment without requisite skills or experience. The group had been initiated by another nurse, who co-led the first few sessions with one of the women. Thus new ties were grafted onto Mary's network through a group-level intervention. Shelley was linked with another child of divorced parents by the school nurse. The school nurse was the catalyst for a buddy system in the local high school. Thus new supportive ties were introduced to Shelley's network. Finally, the CHN suggested that Sean could benefit from referral to a social skills class in his nursery school for children who had difficulty communicating with others. In Sean's case, stuttering and displacement were factors in his communication problems. This individual-level intervention focused on social skills, but had implications for Sean's ability to elicit support from peers and others.

Evaluation Phase

The actual outcome of social support interventions is determined through evaluation. If the predicted outcome is not achieved, other variables related to the person or support context may be discovered (Norbeck, 1982). As noted in Chapter 2, support has indirect and direct effects on health outcomes. Social support may either reduce physical and psychological symptoms (Rook & Dooley, 1985) or contribute more directly to global life-satisfaction or specific well-being states (Pearlin, Lieberman, Managhan, & Mullin, 1981; Ward, 1985). Thus improvements in functioning, health status, and morale are commonly cited outcomes.

Nurse researchers have focused upon buffering effects rather than examining the main effects of social support (see Chapter 5), a problem observed by Thoits (1982). Affective measures clearly predominate in the nursing literature. Main or buffering effects on physical health outcomes are rarely considered. Clearly, physiological outcomes and main, or direct, effects might be increasingly incorporated if primary-prevention interventions are instituted. Nevertheless, Kaplan and Toshima (1990) found few systematic studies of the impact of support interventions on health behaviors and positive health outcomes.

As illustrated in the examples cited in the preceding section, evaluation of social support interventions should focus on outcomes such as enhanced coping, decreased loneliness, situational versus dispositional attributions regarding causes of problems, impact on help seeking from the natural network, reciprocity of supportive interactions, and effects of downward and upward social comparison. It is necessary to document positive and negative impact (such as conflict) on individual members at all levels of interventions. A cost-benefit analysis is imperative. It is important to elicit information from all lay participants (i.e., providers and recipients) regarding perceived needs, use of support, and barriers to such utilization. Finally, the level of satisfaction with quality as well as quantity of potential and actual support should be elicited.

It is noteworthy that although the nursing literature suggests evaluation of group interventions, most reported studies do not use formal research techniques. Informal evaluation by nurses of continuation of groups (Alley & Foster, 1990), impact on behavior and emotion (Halm, 1990), member satisfaction and attendance (Platt, 1990), and comfort voicing complaints and compliance (Sanfilippo et al., 1989) predominate. Evaluation could take the form of questionnaires following group closure, interviews of former group members, indirect measures of continuing mutual aid and self-help, and more formal comparative evaluation with social groups along specific dimensions (Lee, 1988). Evaluation of other levels of support interventions also could examine impact on particular outcomes, as well as delineating process.

Interventions may have mixed effects. Hence the risks and benefits of groups and other interventions should be evaluated. Gottlieb (1988a) recommends monitoring immediate and delayed side effects of interventions, assessing whether gains from interventions are maintained over time, and pre- and post-test measure of support as well as some outcome variable(s) in intervention research. Yet few studies have evaluated long-term effects of support interventions (Bass, Bowman, & Noelker, 1991).

> The evaluation of the outcomes of these support interventions was predominantly positive. Mary's coping and her sense of self-efficacy and self-esteem were enhanced, while her loneliness and social isolation diminished. Eventually she found a satisfying, stable job working with a telephone company that encourages career development and continuing education. She learned how to handle conflicts with her estranged husband now that she no longer felt so dependent on him for financial security. Furthermore, Mary formed friendships at work and in the new neighborhood. Shelley was pleased to have found a friend who not only understood what it was like to be in a single-parent

household, but also introduced her to other boys and girls in her age group. Shelley's newfound popularity among her peers enhanced her self-esteem and led to her election as class president. Sean learned to cope with his stuttering. He enjoyed playing with other children at the nursery school located on his street and was learning to read out loud. Mary's mother no longer had to provide day-to-day practical support. Her sense of burden decreased and she now had time to resume her own friendships and to join a senior citizen's club. Thus Mary's natural network was enhanced and supplemented through nursing support intervention and mutual aid with peers.

Social Support in Nursing Practice Sites

The intervention strategies exemplified in the preceding section reflect practice in the two settings in which nurses practice: the hospital and the community.

Hospital

Several authors discuss the importance of active involvement of family members by hospital-based nurses. Patients interviewed by Simpson (1991) believed that nurses should assist families and patients to cope with the critical-illness experience, provide a supportive visiting environment for families, and include families in patients' interactions with health-care personnel. Sirles and Selleck (1989) suggest that nurses in acute-care settings can ease the emotional stress of families, facilitate caregiving by families when appropriate, and help them identify other sources of support before their transition to the community. Nurses should be concerned about patients with low social support who have no visitors, rather than viewing visitors as a nuisance (Dean, 1989). Nurses can help family members evaluate whether their goals for the patient's recovery are attainable and mobilize support for the critical-illness event (Halm, 1990).

Others have examined interventions pertaining to specific populations, which serve to illustrate the realm of possible target groups for hospital nurses and the potential generalizability of these strategies. Families of critically ill trauma patients are invited to weekly multidisciplinary intervention-planning meetings (Boettcher & Schiller, 1990). A multidisciplinary perinatal support service offers grief counseling to families of stillborns (Pasquarello, 1990). Families of inpatients in rehabilitation units receive information about medical issues and discharge planning (Glennon & Smith, 1990). Nurses conduct presurgery classes for women coping with hysterectomies, provide information and support during hospitalization, and offer a post-discharge support group (Dulaney, Crawford, & Turner, 1990). Group discussion with psycho-educational content provides opportunity for pre-operative patients to discuss fears and to receive information (Lindeman, 1988), yet gaps in practice are evident. Regrettably, hospital nurses in one study did not refer new mothers to volunteer community-support services (Field & Renfrew, 1991).

Community

Nursing authors examine the importance of the nursing role with respect to a variety of community-based groups, most of which comprise people who have chronic conditions or are caregivers. Ambulatory-care centers provide opportunity for nurses to give emotional support and information to cancer patients and their families and to refer to support programs, including transition services, home care, and camps (Anderson, 1989). Community nurses should respond to cardiac patient and family concerns, provide guidance and education, and intervene regarding assessed support deficits (Fridland, Liddell, & Larsson, 1989; Sirles & Selleck, 1989; Stewart & Gregor, 1984). For example, wives of men who had suffered a myocardial infarction wanted support and advice once the patient was back home, through support groups and counseling (Thompson & Cordle, 1988). An 8-week education and support program for newly diagnosed cardiac clients and their families was implemented by nurses in eastern Canada (Wiggins, 1989).

Group support measures are very helpful to caregivers of the elderly (Riffle, 1989) and of other populations. Caregivers of mentally impaired elders, who provide care over extended periods and have low social support, are at high risk for distress or depression. Nursing intervention strategies that offer tangible and emotional support, perhaps mobilized from the caregivers' network, were recommended (Baillie, Norbeck, & Barnes, 1988). As mothers are the key caregivers for chronically ill children, they require supportive intervention (Anderson & Elfert, 1989; Hirose & Ueda, 1990).

Support education programs for adolescents can be implemented by community health nurses. Nurses can include a diabetic teenager's friends in teaching sessions and can link her or his mother with a mutual-aid group (Dean, 1989). Olds, Henderson, Tatelbaum, and Chamber (1988) designed a program to mobilize social support by having a nurse visit low socioeconomic-status teenagers having their first child. The intervention included parenting and health education; recruited support of boyfriends, family, and other friends; and linked the family to community-health and social-service agencies. Positive effects for mother and infant were reported, such as improved health behavior and improved interaction with children (Olds & Kitzman, 1990).

Social support interventions, such as those identified above for adolescents, can be considered primary prevention when "offering ongoing feedback and anticipatory guidance and . . . conditioning a sense of reliable alliance in a peer network characterized by mutual effect" (Gottlieb, 1987, p. 4). A mental health clinical nurse specialist can facilitate a preventive coping-skills group for other at-risk adolescents (Puskar, Lamb, & Martsolf, 1990). Community programs also may teach people social skills to reduce loneliness and isolation. Health-promotion strategies can also consist of broad public-education campaigns "designed to spur the formation and maintenance of peer group ties, more focused training programs designed to teach help skills among citizens and caregivers, and stress inoculation programs in groups of peers anticipating exposure to a stressor" (Gottlieb, 1988a), as in prenatal programs. Social support strategies also have been used in secondary and tertiary preventive interventions, in reducing the duration of health problems (Gottlieb, 1987). For example, nurses offer a day of education, celebration, and support for cancer survivors in Cleveland, Ohio (Gambosi & Ulreich, 1990). "The introduction of supportive lay companions who are either social intimates or strangers who befriend others" (Gottlieb, 1988a, p. 13) is a health-protection strategy that helps to counteract stress around crises and transitions such as parenthood, aging, or bereavement. Nurses working in homes, schools, clinics, and community centers can employ these preventive and promotive support strategies.

Nurses in occupational health settings could use support to enable health behavior change and ameliorate workplace stressors. Partner and group support in smoking-cessation and weight-loss programs (Cohen, 1988) and support training programs for the unemployed (Heller, Price, & Hogg, 1990) could be adapted as support interventions by occupational health nurses.

Occupational Support for Nurses

The theoretical framework of work stress developed by La Rocco et al. (1980) and House (1981) illustrates how social support modifies the relationship between perceived job stress and mental and physical health. Similarly, Israel, Schurman, and House (1989) conceptualize occupational stress as a process that includes a number of moderating factors such as social support on health outcomes. Occupational support protects workers from adverse mental and physical health consequences of job stressors and influences coping with these stressors (Gottlieb, 1982b; La Rocco et al., 1980). A model tested by Dignam & West (1988) revealed that job-site support influenced positive health only through its direct, negative effect on burnout symptoms. Conversely, spillover of stress from work can alter the balance of social relationships (Eckenrode & Gore, 1990).

Nursing studies (e.g., Norbeck, 1985d) demonstrate that these models can be applied to human services. Several studies reveal an association of social support and components of burnout or health. Perceived availability of support was linked with reduced emotional exhaustion/burnout (Firth et al., 1986), and emotional and appraisal support and duration of relationships were inversely related to nursing burnout (Cronin-Stubbs & Rooks, 1985). Interestingly, medical and surgical nurses with numerous sources of support and high levels of satisfaction reported less burnout regardless of level of work stress (Ogus, 1990). Jennings (1990) discovered direct negative effects of social support (not buffering effects) on psychological symptoms of head nurses.

Sources of support have differing effects. Ninety percent of support for 101 community health nurses came from relatives, friends, and work associates; perceived lack of supervisor support was a major stressor (Stewart, 1992). Fong's (1990) investigation of nurse educators discovered that support from work colleagues was significantly and negatively related to depersonalization, whereas supervisor support correlated with sense of accomplishment. The extent to which nursing staff could count on help from coworkers influenced their attitudes about their jobs, affected their health, and enhanced their self-esteem and motivation (Browner, 1987). Chiriboga, Jenkins, and Bailey (1983) found that nurses who perceived their spouses and other staff to be supportive seemed to have the most favorable coping outcomes. Supervisor behavior and work-group relations directly influence role perception among nurses; role ambiguity in turn was linked to decreased job satisfaction (Revicki & May, 1989). Coworker interdependence and relationships help promote the fit between nurses and their work environments (Mansfield, Yu, McLeod, Vickary, & Packard, 1989) and enhance job satisfaction (McCloskey, 1990).

There have been several calls in the nursing literature for increased levels of social support for the stressors in the nursing work situation (e.g., Lindsey & Attridge, 1989), and for alleviation of alienation associated with burnout (Harris, 1989). Nurses may wish to augment social support resources to cope with job stressors in stressful times. For example, work-support groups, mentors, participatory decision making, conflict resolution, programs and policies to enhance the quality of work life, team building, and stress-management techniques are pertinent (Cohen, 1990; Hirsch & David, 1983; Israel et al., 1989; Pasacreta & Jacobsen, 1989; Vance, 1990). Thus support has an impact on job satisfaction, burnout, and health of nurses. Support interventions may be necessary.

Summary

Nurses play numerous indirect support roles (e.g., consultant, facilitator, educator, liaison, and referral agent) and direct surrogate support roles in a variety of hospital and community settings with diverse population groups. Interventions can be at the individual, dyadic, group, community, and social-system levels. Evaluation of outcomes and clear delineation of intervention processes, however, are needed. Finally, support has an impact not only on the health and health behavior of nursing clients but also on nurses experiencing occupational stresses.

❖ CHAPTER FIVE ❖

Nurses' Research Contributions

Nurse researchers have contributed to the conceptualization, measurement, and empirical study of support resources and target populations to the social support literature. This review emphasizes empirical studies rather than the numerous descriptive reports of projects and programs that purportedly involve social support but appear to lack a research base. Only those written by nurses as primary or secondary authors were examined.

Target Populations

Nurse investigators contribute to the social support literature, primarily through research with clinical populations encountered in nursing practice (Norbeck, 1988b). Gottlieb (1987) observes that "as research on the topic of social support accumulates, adding greater precision to our knowledge of the contribution to health made by personal relationships, more attention is being paid to practical application of this knowledge on behalf of clinical and community populations." A review of target populations identified in 63

AUTHOR'S NOTE: This chapter is based on an earlier review reported in three articles, in *Nursing Research* (Stewart, 1989c) and *International Journal of Nursing Research* (Stewart, 1989d, 1989e), of research conducted by nurses prior to 1987 and a more recent search for research reports and instruments published between 1987 and 1991 inclusive.

empirical studies of social support conducted by nurses prior to 1987 is outlined briefly, and the review of the 62 investigations over the past 5 years is delineated in greater detail.

The nursing research targeted for study those who have experienced chronic changes that have long-term effects on social networks and social resources (namely, the physically ill and caregivers) and acute stressful life events. Social support is associated with serious physical illness (Berkman, 1985) in that "illness creates tensions and instigates social losses and estrangements, and network disruptions and dislocations increase vulnerability to illness" (Gottlieb, 1985a). It is indeed appropriate that nurse researchers address these statistically non-normative events, which, according to Schulz and Rau (1985), tend to be less predictable and more stressful. These are situational rather than maturational stressors.

Chronic Situational Stressors: Chronically Ill and Caretaker Populations

Chronic Illness or Disability

The nursing social-support literature, not unexpectedly, emphasized the chronically ill who suffer from physical problems such as a stroke, arthritis, paraplegia (Dixon, 1981), quadriplegia, CVA (McNett, 1987), hemodialysis (Dimond, 1979), cancer (Lindsey, Dodd, & Chen, 1985; Mishel & Braden, 1987; Saunders & McCorkle, 1987), myocardial infarction (Hilbert, 1985), and "medical" illnesses (Ahmadi, 1985; Gardner & Wheeler, 1987). Intuitively, these are appropriate foci of study for this profession, which has ongoing contact with high-risk groups in hospital and community sites.

Since 1987, 11 studies have been conducted that focus on persons with cancer (Bruera, Kuehn, Emery, MacMillan, & Hanson, 1990; Cawley, Kostic, & Cappello, 1990; Hanucharurnkul, 1989), coronary artery disease (Christopherson-Yates, 1989), myocardial infarction (Miller, McMahon, & Garrett, 1989), rheumatoid arthritis (Lambert, Lambert, Klipple, & Mewshaw, 1989), and multiple sclerosis (Foote, Piazza, & Holcombe, 1990); the physically disabled (Birkel & Jones, 1989; McNett, 1987); and the chronically ill (Primono, Yates, & Woods, 1990; Raatikainen, 1991). All studies deal with adult populations, although only 1 includes partners (Christopherson-Yates,

1989). Table 5.1A summarizes the design and outcome of these recent investigations.

Sample sizes range from 40 to 178. Eight studies were correlational and three were descriptive. Most were quantitative, two were qualitative, and one used a combination of approaches. Ten used a cross-sectional design and one used a retrospective approach.

Only McNett (1987) explicitly invokes coping theory as a framework for her study. Two projects are based on nursing theories, specifically Orem's (1980) Self-Care Theory and Kim's (1983a) Model for Collaborative Decision Making. Foote et al. (1990) refer generally to hope and self-esteem constructs without incorporating a theoretical framework.

Five studies found a positive buffering effect of support in the presence of stress on coping effectiveness (Lambert et al., 1989), family functioning (Primono et al., 1990), physical and mental well-being (Raatikainan, 1991), psychosocial well-being (Christopherson-Yates, 1989), and self-care and stage of cancer (Hanucharurnkul, 1989). However, only two studies employ stress measures. Five studies used established social support measures. One study found a negative direct effect on emotion-focused coping and a positive direct effect on problem-focused coping.

Caregivers

Another category of chronic stressors studied, prior to 1987, were the social support needs and networks of the caretakers of the disabled and the ill, such as mothers of children with developmental delays (Brandt, 1984a), parents of children with cancer (Friedman, 1985), children of aged parents (Fuller & Larson, 1980), spouses of individuals with multiple sclerosis (Brandt & Weinert, 1981), families who cared for patients with cancer (Hinds, 1985), and wives of patients admitted to teaching hospitals (Bramwell & Whall, 1986).

Over the past 5 years, studies pertaining to the support needs of these supporters have proliferated. Sixteen investigations have focused on caregivers of adults with physical and mental impairment (Baillie et al., 1988), of adults experiencing surgery (Halm, 1990; Lindsey-Davis, 1990), of adults with Alzheimer's disease (Robinson, 1990), of adults with multiple medical diagnoses (Lindgren, 1990), of stroke survivors (Printz-Fedderson, 1990), of myocardial infarction

(text continued on page 116)

Table 5.1 Target Populations in Nursing Literature on Social Support (SS), 1987-1991

Study	*Sample*	*Design*	*Theoretical Framework*	*Stress Measure*	*Support Measure*	*Other Variables*	*Effect/Outcomes Main*	*Effect/Outcomes Buffering*	*Results*
A. CHRONIC CONDITIONS									
Birkel & Jones (1989)	20 cognitively impaired and physically disabled elders, 20 physically disabled elders	Cross-sectional, correlational, quantitative	—	—	Helper Network Interview (assesses size, composition, and quality of network)	1. Mental Status Assessment 2. Mental Status Questionnaire 3. Face Hand Test 4. Physical Health Status Rating 5. The Long-Term Care Information Assessment Process	—	—	Dementia is a critical determinant of network size and composition
Bruera et al. (1990)	169 consecutive admissions to a palliative care unit	Retrospective, descriptive	—	—	Question assessing the number of support persons within and outside the household	Demographics	—	—	Lack of family support and lack of intensive home care services are the main obstacles to home care for terminally ill cancer patients
Cawley et al. (1990)	68 women with early-stage breast cancer	Cross-sectional, descriptive, quantitative-qualitatitive	—	—	3 questions related to support needs	Interview questions related to information and physical needs	—	—	Support needs met in terms of family and friends; needs expressed for support groups

Christopherson-Yates (1989)	94 males with coronary artery disease and 85 partners	Cross-sectional, correlational, qualitative	—	Questions developed for study concerning stress level	Questions developed for study about SS system	Psychological well-being assessed by interview questions	Nonsupportive exchanges lead to stress	Increase of partner support on psychological well-being of patients and decrease stress	Greater levels of psychological and relational well-being associated with greater age, less change, less stress, and less partner hindrance
Foote et al. (1990)	40 adults with multiple sclerosis	Cross-sectional, correlational, quantitative	—	—	Personal Resource Questionnaire Part 2	1. Miller Hope Scale 2. Rosenberg Self-Esteem Scale	—	Social support related to hope and to self-esteem	Individuals with a higher level of hope perceived higher self-esteem and social support
Hanucharurnkul (1989)	112 adult cervical & head/neck cancer patients	Cross-sectional, correlational, quantitative	Orem (1985) Self-Care Model	—	Social Support Questionnaire NSSQ	1. Self-Care Behavior Questionnaire 2. Quality of Life Index 3. Cantril Ladder Scale	—	On the relationship between stage and site of cancer and self-care	Social support and SES are strong predictors of self-care
Lambert et al. (1989)	122 women with rheumatoid arthritis	Cross-sectional, correlational, quantitative	—	—	Social Support Measure (Sarason et al., 1983)	1. Mental Health Index 2. Keitel Functional Test 3. Morning Stiffness 4. Sedimentation Rate 5. Kobcoa Hardiness Measure	—	On the coping effectiveness for women with arthritis	Social support and hardiness are significant predictors of psychological well-being regardless of severity of illnesses

(Continued)

Table 5.1 (Continued)

Study	Sample	Design	*Theoretical Framework*	*Stress Measure*	*Support Measure*	*Other Variables*	*Effect/Outcomes*		Results
							Main	*Buffering*	
McNett (1987)[b]	50 wheelchair-bound adults	Cross-sectional, correlational, quantitative	Coping (Lazarus & Folkman, 1984)	—	Interpersonal Support Evaluation List Questions concerning support effectiveness	1. Ways of Coping Checklist, 2. McNett Coping Effectiveness Questionnaire	Negative direct effect on emotion-focused coping and a positive direct effect on problem-focused coping	—	—
Miller et al. (1989)	50 postmyocardial infarction patients	Cross-sectional, descriptive, qualitative	—	—	Questions concerning sources of support	—	—	—	Patients were the greatest positive supporters of themselves; family and friends EC & TS; health team perceived as negative and ambiguous
Primomo et al. (1990)	125 chronically ill women	Cross-sectional, correlational, quantitative	—	Demands of Illness Inventory	Norbeck Social Support Questionnaire	FACES-II Spanier Dyadic Adjustment Scale CES-D (Center for Epidemiological Studies-Depression)	—	Affective support from friends and reciprocity related to family functioning	A greater perception of affect and affirmation from spouse and family related to greater marital quality, family functioning, and lower illness demands and depression
Rautikainen (1991)	178 patients in domiciliary care	Cross-sectional, correlational, quantitative	Kim (1983) Model of Decision Making	—	Questions developed for study concerning social support	Reports of physical and mental well-being	—	On physical and emotional well-being	Support of relatives in care related to patients, ability to cope

B. CAREGIVERS

Baillie et al. (1988)	87 caregivers of physically and mentally impaired adults	Cross-sectional, correlational, quantitative	House (1981)	Profile of Mood States, Perceived Stress of Caregiving (16 items)	8 questions developed for this study assessing satisfaction with support	Psychological Distress and Depression (interview questions) 19% 22% variance	Main effect for social support in predicting psychological distress	No buffering effects; social support decreases, increased burdens lead to distress and depression	There were main effects of perceived stress and satisfaction with social support on psychological distress and depression
Capuzzi (1989)	15 mothers of physically handicapped children, 21 mothers of children with no handicaps	Longitudinal, correlational	—	—	Norbeck Social Support Questionnaire	Nursing Child Assessment Feeding Scale	—	Maternal attachment buffers stress of having MC infant	Presence of social support affirmation reduces the stress, facilitating maternal attachment
Clements et al. (1990)	30 families of children with diabetes, cancer, or cystic fibrosis	Cross-sectional qualitative, descriptive (interview)	—	Questions concerning stress associated with caregiving	Questions concerning support needs	—	—	—	When emotional and physical support is available to meet family needs, equilibrium is achieved
Florian & Krulik (1991)	90 mothers of children with cancer, cystic fibrosis, diabetes, or epilepsy; 92 mothers of healthy children	Cross-sectional, correlational, quantitative	Loneliness	—	Norbeck Social Support Questionnaire	UCLA Loneliness Scale, social network size and amount of support	—	Absence of formal support sources	Mothers of chronically ill children experience higher feelings of loneliness than mothers of healthy children; mothers of children with life-threatening diseases report larger social networks and perceive greater support

(*Continued*)

Table 5.1 (Continued)

Study	*Sample*	*Design*	*Theoretical Framework*	*Stress Measure*	*Support Measure*	*Other Variables*	*Effect/Outcomes* *Main*	*Buffering*	*Results*
Geary (1989)	20 mothers who were monitoring apneic infants	Longitudinal, qualitative-quantitative, descriptive	—	Interview questions concerning stress levels	1. Inventory of Socially Supportive Behaviors 2. Norbeck Social Support questionnaire	—	—	—	Interview schedule identified 10 major themes: discussions with others, resolve, possible death of the baby, why this happened, demands & changes, adjusting to monitor, managing the monitor, and time perspectives
Halm (1990)[c]	30 family caregivers of adults experiencing surgery with bedside support, 25 caregivers involved in a support group	Quasi-experimental, quantitative	Crisis Theory (Caplan, 1964)	—	—	State-Trait Anxiety Inventory	—	Anxiety	Experimental subjects had a significant reduction in anxiety from pre-measures to post-measures
Hirose & Ueda (1990)	28 mothers and fathers of children with cerebral palsy	Cross-sectional (interviews), descriptive, qualitative	—	—	Interview questions concerning support network	Interview questions concerning social, mental, and physical condition of parents and acceptance of situation	—	—	The most helpful persons for mothers and fathers were their spouses or support source

Lindgren (1990)	51 family caregivers of adults with multiple medical diagnoses	Cross-sectional, correlational, quantitative	Coping (Lazarus, 1984)	—	Norbeck Social Support Questionnaire	Maslach Burnout Inventory	—	Burnout, emotion, exhaustion, and social support slightly	Social support measures of affect and affirmation modified burnout as depersonalization whereas affirmation and aid related to personal accomplishment
Lindsey-Davis (1990)	109 recovering individuals and their family caregivers	Cross-sectional, correlational, quantitative	—	Lefebvre and Sanford Multimodel Stress Questionnaire	Personal Resource Questionnaire (social support potential, use of potential network scales)	Mishel Illness Uncertainty Scale	Illness uncertainty	—	Uncertainty was related to lower perceived social support potential and reduced use of the network for family caregivers
MacCarthy (1989)	45 caregivers of adults attending a day hospital for psychiatric disorder	Cross-sectional (interview), descriptive, qualitative-quantitative	—	—	Questions developed for this study concerning quantity and quality of social contacts	Social Behavior Schedule Interview questions concerning objective burden	—	—	The patients' disturbed behavior and functional deficits appeared to impose a strain on the supporters' mental health rather than their social and economic well-being
McCubbin (1989)	27 single-parent families and 27 two-parent families of children with cerebral palsy	Cross-sectional, correlational, quantitative	Typology Model of Adjustment and Adaptation (McCubbin & McCubbin, 1987)	Family Inventory of Life Events (section on stressors)	Family Inventory of Resources for Management (extended family support)	Physical Health Status, Overall Health Improvement, CHIP, Family Adaptability and Cohesion, Evaluation Scales	—	—	No significant differences in family stress between single-parent and two-parent families

(Continued)

Table 5.1 (Continued)

Study	*Sample*	*Design*	*Theoretical Framework*	*Stress Measure*	*Support Measure*	*Other Variables*	*Effect/Outcomes* *Main*	*Buffering*	*Results*
Norbeck (1991a)	60 family caregivers of child, adult, and elderly psychiatric patients	Cross-sectional, descriptive, qualitative-quantitative (interview)	—	—	Interview guide assessing support needs based on current problems, hypothesized situations	—	—	Need for respite, social contact, companionship	Support needs expressed parallel general support categories: emotional, feedback, informational, and instrumental
Printz-Fedderson (1990)[c]	21 stroke survivors with known caregivers, 17 stroke survivors whose caregivers attended a support group	Ex post facto study, quantitative	—	—	—	CADET Physical Caregiving Responsibility Inventory, The Geriatric Depression Scale	—	—	Advanced educational status, high income, and moderate physical disabilities were related to reduced feelings of burden; there were no significant differences between the two groups
Robinson (1990)	31 adult caregivers of adults with Alzheimer's disease and related disorders	Cross-sectional, correlational, quantitative	Tolsdorf (1976)	—	Norbeck Social Support Questionnaire, Sarason's Social Support Questionnaire	—	Self-esteem	AAA increased and SE increased; SN less increase and SE decreased	Significant positive relationships between social skills and available support and between functional social support and self-esteem

Sterling (1990)	19 mothers and 1 grandmother of infants with chronic lung disease	Cross-sectional (interview), descriptive, qualitative	—	—	Questions developed for study concerning support needs	—	—	—	Parents utilized a variety of resources and reported needs in the areas of knowledge/ skills, time, material resources, and support
Thompson (1988)	76 wives of patients suffering first myocardial infarction	Cross-sectional (questionnaire), descriptive, qualitative	—	—	Questions concerning support received	—	—	—	Caregivers felt they were poorly informed about myocardial infarction, had little opportunity for expert information, and had received most support from relatives
C. ACUTE: CRITICAL ILLNESS/SURGERY									
Northouse (1988)	50 breast cancer patients hospitalized for first mastectomy	Cross-sectional, correlational, descriptive	House (1981)	—	Social Support Questionnaire	Affects Balance Scale, Brief Symptom Inventory, Psychosocial Adjustment to Illness	On adjustment	—	Patients and husbands who reported higher levels of combined support from family, friends, nurses, and physicians reported fewer adjustment problems

(Continued)

Table 5.1 (Continued)

Study	*Sample*	*Design*	*Theoretical Framework*	*Stress Measure*	*Support Measure*	*Other Variables*	*Effect/Outcomes Main*	*Effect/Outcomes Buffering*	*Results*
D. ACUTE: STRESSFUL SITUATION: ABUSE									
Henderson (1989)	8 physically abused women in the process of leaving the relationship	Cross-sectional, qualitative (interview), descriptive; interviews 10 days, 1 month, and 2 months after leaving transition house	—	—	Questions concerning relationships, social isolation, and plans for the future	—	—	—	Quality of support received had a major influence on ability to adapt to their situations; social support process/ stages: reassurance, analysis, reciprocity, independence
E. PREGNANCY AND NEW PARENTHOOD									
Aaronson (1989)[d]	529 pregnant women	Cross-sectional, correlational, quantitative	—	—	1. Personal Resource Questionnaire 2. Questions concerning perceived and received support	Data on adherence to health behaviors (alcohol, caffeine, and cigarettes)	—	On promoting positive health behaviors	Received and perceived support may act differently with respect to buffering stress and promoting positive health behaviors; those who lived with a smoker perceived less general and specific support for not smoking

Albrecht & Rankin (1989)[d]	47 pregnant women (various SES, races, and religions)	Cross-sectional, correlational, descriptive, quantitative	—	—	Personal Resource Questionnaire	Health Behavior Questionnaire, State-Trait Anxiety Inventory	—	Anxiety	Lack of support is associated with increased state-trait anxiety levels and consumption of alcohol
Boyce et al. (1988)	5 unmarried, adolescent, pregnant women	Longitudinal, descriptive, qualitative (interview)	—	—	Interview questions designed for study concerning support network	—	—	—	Women who had successfully accommodated to life as a teenage parent had more detailed and differentiated views of their network; adaptive capacity flexible, broad, perceived support functions
Dormire et al. (1989)	18 adolescent first-time mothers	Cross-sectional, correlational, descriptive, quantitative	Coping (Lazarus & Folkman, 1984)	Parenting Stress Index	Norbeck Social Support Questionnaire	Nursing Child Assessment Teaching Scale (NCATS)	—	Total functional SS not significantly related to stress	Social support and parent-infant interaction reciprocity were positively related

(Continued)

Table 5.1 (Continued)

Study	*Sample*	*Design*	*Theoretical Framework*	*Stress Measure*	*Support Measure*	*Other Variables*	*Effect/Outcomes Main*	*Effect/Outcomes Buffering*	*Results*
Ferketich & Mercer (1990)[c]	87 high-risk pregnant women and 139 low-risk pregnant women	Cross-sectional correlational, quantitative	—	Negative Life Events Survey, Pregnancy Risk Score, Intrapartal Risk Score	1. Inventory of socially supportive behaviors 2. Checklist of supportive persons 3. 6-item scale on perceived support	1. General Health Index 2. Self-Esteem Scale 3. Sense of Mastery 4. Parental Sense of Competence 5. Trait Anxiety Inventory 6. Center for Epidemiologic Studies Depression Scale 7. Feetham Family Functioning Survey 8. Marital Adjustment Test	—	On health status	Stress from negative life events had small indirect effects on health status through self-esteem, parental competence, family functioning, mate relationship, and perceived support
Kaufman & Hall (1989)	125 mothers of preterm infants	Longitudinal (9 mos.) qualitative, prospective, analytic	—	—	Influence of Specific Referents Scale—perception of network influence; Social Network Support—number of referents providing support	Breast-feeding choice and duration were recorded	—	—	The mother's perception of influence from referents and number of supports in her network predicted choice to breast-feed or bottle-feed; women with no source of support were more likely to cease breast-feeding; husband or partner support reported by 75%

McHaffie (1989)	21 mothers of very-low-birthweight babies	Longitudinal interviews at 6 occasions; descriptive, qualitative-quantitative	—	—	Questions concerning sources of help and quality of help	Neonatal Perception Inventory, Demographic Diaries	—	—	Family can be a strong source of support in times of crisis but they do not often release appropriate forms of help; partner supportive; mother most supportive after delivery but then diminishes; relatives unsupportive; conflicting advice and information given
Norbeck & Anderson (1989a)[d]	208 low-income pregnant women (African-American, Hispanic, and white)	Longitudinal (mid & late pregnancy), correlational, quantitative	—	Revised Life Events Questionnaire	Norbeck Social Support Questionnaire	1. Spielberger State-Trait Anxiety Inventory 2. Substance Use Complications 3. Birth weights 4. Gestational ages	—	—	Lack of significance for life stress and anxiety in predicting pregnancy outcomes as well as for stress-support interactions; for African-American women, partner or mother support accounted for 33% of pregnancy complications; for white women, high rather than low SS accounted for pregnancy outcomes and substance abuse (i.e., reinforce negative health practices)

(Continued)

Table 5.1 (Continued)

Study	*Sample*	*Design*	*Theoretical Framework*	*Stress Measure*	*Support Measure*	*Other Variables*	*Effect/Outcomes Main*	*Effect/Outcomes Buffering*	*Results*
Norbeck & Anderson (1989b)	190 low-income women (African-American, Hispanic, and white)	Longitudinal, quantitative, correlational (prospective time, 1-17-26 weeks, gestational 2-32-40 weeks)	—	Revised Life Events Questionnaire	Norbeck Social Support Questionnaire	State-Trait Anxiety Inventory	—	On level of anxiety	Life stress, social support, and anxiety are stable from mid- to late pregnancy; high anxiety related to high stress/low support and low anxiety related to low stress/high support (explained 30%–40% of variance); combination of high stress and low partner support with high anxiety
Richardson (1987)	30 women who experienced premature labor and 15 women with normal pregnancies	Longitudinal, qualitative (interviews)	—	—	Interview Schedule Questions involving important relationships and the changes or problems associated with these relationships (face validity and reliability of 94)	—	—	—	Premature labor subjects reported significantly more unsatisfactory/problematic relationships with important persons (husbands and parental figures in particular); 55% of relationships satisfactory compared to 85% for those with normal pregnancies—less help and affection

F. AGING									
Beatty-Nelson (1989)	26 institutionalized elderly people without history of depression	Cross-sectional, correlational, quantitative	Stress-illness model (Selye, 1956)	—	Norbeck Social Support Questionnaire	Geriatric Depression Scale, Rosenberg's Self-esteem Scale	—	—	Social support was significantly correlated with depression; mean # in social network was 9.12; Moderate correlations between self-esteem and all components of social support
G. DETERIORATION OF THE NETWORK: DIVORCE									
Duffy (1989)	72 divorced women with custody of 1 or more children under 18	Cross-sectional, quantitative (interview), descriptive		—	Semi-structured interview guide, four questions asking about types of support, primary support person, and distinguishing features	—	—	—	Qualities of continuity, availability, and understanding in primary support persons allowed relationships to transcend life changes associated with divorce; women named other women as primary support sources; four groups of primary support: ex-spouse/lover, relative, friend/work associate, and neighbor

(Continued)

Table 5.1 (Continued)

Study	*Sample*	*Design*	*Theoretical Framework*	*Stress Measure*	*Support Measure*	*Other Variables*	*Effect/Outcomes* *Main*	*Buffering*	*Results*
H. HEALTH PROMOTION AND PREVENTION									
Aaronson (1989)	529 pregnant women	Cross-sectional, correlational, quantitative	—	—	1. Personal Resource Questionnaire 2. Questions concerning perceived and received support	Data on adherence to health behaviors (alcohol, caffeine, and cigarettes)	—	On promoting health behaviors	Received and perceived support may act differently with respect to buffering stress and promoting positive health behaviors; those who lived with a smoker perceived less specific support for not smoking
Albrecht & Rankin (1989)	47 pregnant women (variety of SES, races, and religions)	Cross-sectional, correlational, descriptive, quantitative	—	—	Personal Resource Questionnaire	1. Health Behavior Questionnaire 2. State-Trait Anxiety Inventory	—	Anxiety	Lack of support is associated with increased state-trait anxiety levels and consumption of alcohol
Boyle (1989)	53 men and women from an urban community in El Salvador	Cross-sectional, qualitative, descriptive (interview), ethnographic	—	Questions concerning stress management	Interview questions concerning social support and social network and participant observation	Observation and calendar records of exercise, nutrition, and weight control	—	Well-being	Availability of family members, social networks, and religious and community support promotes the adoption of health-enhancing behaviors and appears to be an important determinant of health promotion beliefs and practices

Gonzalez (1990)	106 low-income Mexican-American women attending a health clinic	Cross-sectional, descriptive	—	—	Ratings of support from 5 most important people and 9 items assessing perceptions of health-related emotional and material support	1. 5 items assessing barriers to health care 2. English language proficiency 3. 11 items related to self-efficacy-BSF 4. Frequency of breast self-examination	—	Health	Utilization barriers to health care can be softened by the presence of high self-efficacy; lack of association between social support and behavior in scale and self-efficacy (may be due to scale)
Jacobson (1990)	85 normal adolescents	Cross-sectional, correlational, quantitative	Depression Theories (Beck, 1967; Langmeier & Matejcek, 1975) and Weiss (1975) Theory of Social Support	—	Personal Resource Questionnaire Part 2	Beck Depression inventory	On depression	—	Moderate statistically significant inverse relationship between social support and depression
Norbeck & Anderson (1989a)	190 low-income women (African-American, Hispanic, and white)	Longitudinal, quantitative, correlational (prospective time, 1-17-26 weeks; gestation 2-32-40 weeks)	—	Revised Life Events Questionnaire	Norbeck Social Support Questionnaire	State-Trait Anxiety Inventory	—	Anxiety	Life stress, social support, and anxiety are stable from mid- to late pregnancy; high anxiety related to high stress/low support and low anxiety to low stress/high support and high anxiety (explained 30%–40% of the variance)

(Continued)

Table 5.1 (Continued)

Study	*Sample*	*Design*	*Theoretical Framework*	*Stress Measure*	*Support Measure*	*Other Variables*	*Effect/Outcomes Main*	*Effect/Outcomes Buffering*	*Results*
Riffle et al. (1989)	113 people 55 years or over attending nutrition sites	Cross-sectional, correlational, descriptive	—	Stress management scale from HPLP	1. Interpersonal support scale from the Health Promoting Lifestyle Profile 2. Personal Resources Questionnaire Part 2 (PRQ2)	Health Promoting Lifestyle Profile Scale	—	—	Significant positive correlations of PRQ2 scores (support) with self-actualization, health responsibility, interpersonal support, and stress management
Rutledge (1987)	93 women from a variety of women's groups questioned concerning breast self-examination (BSE)	Cross-sectional, correlational, quantitative	Health Belief Model (Becker, 1974)	—	Norbeck Social Support Questionnaire	Tennessee Self-Concept Scale, modified version of Champion Health Belief Model (1984), number of times BSE practiced in the last year	None found	—	Positive correlation found between self-concept and frequency of BSE; no relation for social support/network properties
Schank & Long (1989)	50 elderly women in private housing and 50 elderly women in public housing	Cross-sectional, qualitative, descriptive (interview)	—	—	Structured 37-item interview designed for study with a section on social support	Interview sections on health status and biographical data	—	—	Excellent or good health status related to greater social support; women in private housing with good health status had a greater degree of social support more frequently than women in public housing

I. OCCUPATIONAL SUPPORT FOR NURSES (FROM 1985)									
Bizek & Oermann (1990)	73 critical care nurse preceptors	Cross-sectional, correlational, descriptive	—	—	25 questions on benefits, rewards, recognition, and sources of guidance	Slavitt Job Satisfaction Scale (48 items)	—	—	Significant positive correlation between perceived work from institution support and level of job satisfaction (in particular organizational requirements, interaction, and job prestige)
Comi-McCloskey (1990)	150 newly employed nurses	Cross-sectional, quantitative, correlational	—	—	Social Integration Measure (8 items, 5-pt. scale)	1. Job Characteristics Inventory 2. 3 items from Job Diagnostic Survey 3. Organizational Commitment Questionnaire 4. Work motivation 5. Intention to stay on job	—	Social integration buffered bad effects of low autonomy	Low perceived autonomy and low perceived social integration associated with low job satisfaction, motivation, and commitment
Cronin-Stubbs & Brophy (1985)	296 nurses in either psychiatry, operating room, intensive care, or medicine specialties	Cross-sectional, correlational, descriptive	—	1. Nursing Stress Scale 2. Life Experience Survey	Norbeck Social Support Questionnaire	Staff Burnout Scale for Health Professionals	—	—	Social support was negatively associated with burnout; affected emotional and affirmational support and duration of relationship, not network size, were negatively related to burnout; frequent interpersonal contacts positively contributed to burnout

(Continued)

Table 5.1 (Continued)

Study	Sample	Design	Theoretical Framework	Stress Measure	Support Measure	Other Variables	Effect/Outcomes Main	Effect/Outcomes Buffering	Results
Cronin-Stubbs & Rooks (1985)	296 nurses in either psychiatry, operating room, intensive care, or medicine specialties	Cross-sectional, correlational, descriptive	—	1. Nursing Stress Scale 2. Life Experience Survey	Norbeck Social Support Questionnaire	Staff Burnout Scale for Health Professionals	—	—	Affect, expressions of liking, admiration, respect, or love predicted burnout (negative association), whereas affirmation or acknowledgment by others did not
Fong (1990)	141 nurse educators	Cross-sectional, correlational, and 35 in-depth interviews	Cherniss (1980) Role overload & La Rocco, House, & French (1980) Model of occupational stress	—	—	1. Maslach Burnout Inventory 2. Moos Work Environment Scale 3. Faculty Activities Survey	—	No buffering effects of SS on overload burnout	Lack of peer support correlated with depersonalization; chairperson support predicted sense of accomplishment, degree of support with burnout
Haberman-Cohen (1990)	43 county public health directors of nursing	Cross-sectional, correlational, quantitative	Model of relationships among stressors, resistance resources (e.g. SS) and outcome of psychological well-being	Revised Hassles and Uplifts Questionnaire (Delongis, 1988), questions on stress	People Around You Scale (emotional and tangible support) interview questions on social support	Brief Symptom Inventory, Life Orientation Test (optimism)	—	—	Coworker support correlated with psychological symptoms; satisfaction with support related to coping; total hassles and coworker support accounted for 6.57% of variance in psychological well-being

Hopkins-Kavanagh (1989)	35 psychiatric nurses	Cross-sectional, qualitative, descriptive	—	—	Network analysis interview developed for this study assessing size and function	—	—	—	Majority of nurses assess their personal relationships as most significant and most supportive and report a desire for more supportive and individualized associations between levels of psychiatric nursing hierarchy
Jennings (1990)	300 head nurses	Cross-sectional, correlational, quantitative-qualitative	—	Administrative Stress Index	Norbeck Social Support Questionnaire, People Around You Scale	1. Brief Symptom Inventory 2. Life Events Questionnaire 3. Locus of Control (Reutter)	On psychological symptoms (weak and negative)	None found; stress and psychological symptoms	Negative correlations between years as a head nurse and psychological symptoms
Kneeshaw (1990)	2,392 nurses responded to a questionnaire identifying 324 smokers	Cross-sectional, quantitative, descriptive	Open Systems Framework (King, 1981)	—	Questionnaire assessing personal data, smoking history, and coworker responses to attempts to quit	—	—	—	Nurses who currently smoke perceive coworkers as more supportive than discouraging
Lindsey & Attridge (1989)	30 acute care nurses returning to university to complete B.Sc. Nursing degrees	Cross-sectional, critical incident technique, qualitative, descriptive	—	—	Questions concerning social support events, the supporter, and perceptions of support and its effects	—	—	—	Nurses who reported unsupportive incidents (e.g., control over work and from physicians) had greatest impact on work performance; felt most supported when the need for acknowledgment of their value and expertise was met

(Continued)

Table 5.1 (Continued)

Study	Sample	Design	Theoretical Framework	Stress Measure	Support Measure	Other Variables	Effect/Outcomes Main	Effect/Outcomes Buffering	Results
Marshall (1989)[a]	161 nursing students	Cross-sectional, qualitative, descriptive	Definition of social support by Schaefer et al. (1981) and definition of dissupport by Malone (1988)	—	Malone Social Network Inventory—assessed network size and perceived helpfulness	—	—	—	Students who dropped out of the nursing program with academic problems were older and had smaller social networks; remaining students gave network members higher ratings of helpfulness, and reported less dissonance between ratings of helpfulness and expectations
Norbeck (1985b)	164 critical care nurses	Cross-sectional, correlational, descriptive	LaRocco et al. (1980) Model of Occupational Stress (adapted and tested)	Questionnaire of Stressful Factors	Norbeck Social Support Questionnaire (modified by addition of 2 situation-specific questions)	1. Nursing Job Satisfaction Scale 2. Brief Symptom Inventory (psychological)	From relatives on perceived job stress and psychological symptoms	None found	Effects of social support were models (4.9% of variance of perceived job stress and 5.4% of variance in psychological symptoms); work support accounted for 7.6% of variance

(Continued)

Ogus (1990)	128 medical and surgical ward nurses	Cross-sectional, quantitative, correlational	—	Nursing Stress Inventory	1. Social Support Questionnaire Short Form 2. Fundy Support Measure	Maslach Burnout Inventory	Amount of satisfaction with SS on burnout	None found	Nurses with high sources of SS and high levels of satisfaction with SS reported less burnout than nurses with few sources of SS and less satisfaction, regardless of level of work stress
Pagana (1990)	246 nursing university and college students	Cross-sectional, qualitative, correlational	Lazarus (1966) and Stress-appraised and Kobasa (1979) Hardiness	Clinical Stress Question-naire (modi-fied from Folkman & Lazarus)	Norbeck Social Support Ques-tionnaire	Third-generation Hardiness Test, 50 items	—	—	Social support was positively related to the evaluation of challenge when using a work-related measure of support but no sig-nificant effect was found between total functional SS and threat and challenge
Skiles & Hinson (1989)	43 nurses, physician assistants, or nurse practition-ers in correctional care setting	Cross-sectional, quantitative, correlational	—	Perceived Stress Scale (14 items)	Inventory of Socially Supportive Behaviors (revised version)	Maslach Burnout Inventory	—	—	Social support was not significantly correlated with any variables except age; as age increased the amount of per-ceived support decreased.

[a] These studies also appear in Table 5.3.
[b] These studies also appear in Table 5.5.
[c] These studies also appear in Table 5.2.
[d] These studies also appear in the Health Promotion and Prevention Section (section H) of Table 5.1.

survivors (Thompson, 1988), of persons with psychiatric disorders (MacCarthy, 1989; Norbeck, 1991b), and of children with chronic physical illnesses (Capuzzi, 1989; Clements, Copeland, & Loftus, 1990; Florian & Krulik, 1991; Geary, 1989; Hirose & Ueda, 1990; McCubbin, 1989; Sterling, 1990) (see Table 5.1B).

Lindgren (1990) explicates a theoretical framework—coping—for her study of burnout and social support in family caregivers. McCubbin (1989) bases her study of families with handicapped children on her own 1987 Typology Model of Adjustment and Adaptation. Loneliness as a construct, although alluded to briefly by Florian and Krulik (1991), was not used as a framework. Robinson (1990) depicted a framework involving social skills, self-esteem, social support, and burden that was based on Tolsdorf's (1976) conceptualization of support. Baillie et al. (1988) employed the stress-buffering model of social support advanced by House (1981). Finally, Halm (1990) called upon crisis theory (Caplan, 1974) as a foundation for her study of caregivers of adults experiencing surgery.

Twelve studies were cross-sectional and two were longitudinal (Capuzzi, 1989; Geary, 1989). Although one was quasi-experimental (Halm, 1990) and one was ex post facto (Printz-Fedderson, 1990), studies were predominantly descriptive or correlational. Five studies used a quantitative design, three combined qualitative and quantitative approaches, and four were qualitative. Seven studies used an established instrument to measure social support—primarily the Norbeck Social Support Questionnaire (discussed in a later section). The remaining studies used questions developed to assess satisfaction with support (e.g., Baillie et al., 1988), quality of social contacts (e.g., MacCarthy et al., 1989; Thompson, 1988), and support needs (e.g., Clements et al., 1990; Norbeck, 1991b; Sterling, 1990) of specific populations or to examine the effects of attending a support group (Halm, 1990; Printz-Fedderson, 1990). Only three studies used an interview approach (Clements et al., 1990; MacCarthy et al., 1989; Sterling, 1990).

Three studies reported a buffering effect on anxiety (Halm, 1990), maternal attachment (Capuzzi, 1989), and burnout (Lindgren, 1990). Three studies found main/direct effects on self-esteem (Robinson, 1990), psychological distress (Baillie et al., 1988), and illness uncertainty (Lindsey-Davis, 1990). Hemophiliacs with AIDS (N=30), family caregivers (N=23), and bereaved caregivers (N=17) encountered absent or negative support, such as avoidance by friends, prejudice from health-care workers and the general community, and the perceived need to preserve confidentiality about the stigmatized illness because of fear of negative reactions (Hart, Mann, & Stewart, 1991).

Acute Situational Stressors: Ill and Abused Populations

As would be expected, some of the focus in the early nursing literature is on individuals who have undergone surgery that may negatively affect their social network and social support, such as hysterectomy (Jackson, 1985; Webb & Wilson-Barnett, 1983), mastectomy (Woods & Earp, 1978), and ostomy (Lucas, 1985). Many of these surgical interventions affect body image and therefore sexual and confiding relationships with spouse or partner. Furthermore, social support can influence rate of recovery from such surgery. More recently Northouse (1988) reported a main effect of social support on patients' and husbands' adjustment to mastectomy (Table 5.1C). Cawley et al. (1990) assessed the informational and psychosocial needs of women with cancer choosing breast-conservation surgery (Table 5.1A).

The social support needs of victims of abuse, another situational stressor or life event, receive little attention in the nursing literature, although McKenna (1985) and Hoff (1985) did examine the social support and/or social networks of battered wives, and Burgess and Holmstrom (1978) studied victims of rape. Henderson (1989) interviewed eight women who had been in violent relationships, at three points in time (10 days, 1 month, and 2 months) after the women left a transition house. This qualitative study reported that quality of relationships with other people in the house influenced adaptation to the transition. The social support process included four stages that progressed from reassurance, to analysis, to reciprocity, and to independence (see Table 5.1D).

Populations Experiencing Maturational Transitions

Life events that actually and potentially involve losses from the social network and those that impose chronic and acute strains on the social network are illustrated in the target populations of empirical nursing studies on social support. Approximately one third of the empirical work focuses on groups that have undergone maturational or developmental life transitions, which inevitably alter the size of the network through birth or death. However, most emphasize the impact of gains through entry of a new member rather than losses through exits.

New Parenthood

Pregnant women (Norbeck & Tilden, 1983; Rich, 1978), expectant couples (Brown, 1986a, 1986b; Cranley, 1984; Zachariah, 1985), and parents of infants (Barnard, Synder, & Spietz, 1984; Cronenwett, 1984, 1985b; Hall, Schaefer, & Greenberg, 1987; Hewat & Ellis, 1984; Jordan, 1985; Lenz, Parks, Jenkins, & Jarrett, 1986; Mercer, Hackley, & Bostrom, 1984; Pridham, 1984; Ventura, 1982) were the foci of earlier studies that examined potential or actual additions to the social network. Although the social network is expanded, strains necessitating supportive interventions from informal and formal sources inevitably accompany new or impending parenthood.

Since 1987, 10 studies have dealt with pregnant women (Aaronson, 1989; Albrecht & Rankin, 1989; Boyce, Kay, & Uitti, 1988; Ferketich & Mercer, 1990; Norbeck & Anderson, 1989a, 1989b), mothers of preterm infants or low-birthweight babies (Kaufman & Hall, 1989; McHaffie, 1989; Richardson, 1987), and adolescent first-time mothers (Dormire, Strauss, & Clarke, 1989) (see Table 5.1E). Boyce et al. (1988) also acknowledge high-risk adolescents in their sampling, and Norbeck and Anderson (1989a, 1989b) consider cultural and economic factors. In contrast to other target populations, there are equal numbers of cross-sectional (5) and longitudinal studies (5). Two studies are correlational and descriptive, five studies are correlational, and three are descriptive. Four investigations employ a qualitative design.

Lazarus and Folkman's (1984) coping theory is invoked by Dormire et al. (1989) but is not measured by a coping instrument. No theoretical frameworks guide the remaining nine studies. Support measures are varied, including the Personal Resources Questionnaire, the NSSQ (these two are discussed in the nursing social-support instrument section), and the Inventory of Socially Supportive Behaviors (an established psychosocial instrument). Others design questions for purposes of the study about the support network (Boyce et al., 1988), and the quality of help or relationships (e.g., McHaffie, 1989; Richardson, 1987). Kaufman and Hall (1989) used their own Influence of Special Referents Scale (Kaufman, 1986) developed to measure a mother's perception of influence from her social network.

The buffering effect of support was demonstrated on health behavior (Aaronson, 1989), anxiety (Albrecht & Rankin, 1989; Norbeck & Anderson, 1989b), and health status (Ferketich & Mercer, 1990). Only four projects incorporated a stress measure. No studies tested the main effect of support. However, support correlated positively with parent-infant interaction and duration of lactation. Peer support was linked with substance abuse in one study, illustrating the negative impact of the network.

Aging Populations

The social-psychological and medical literatures lend credence to the merits of the study of aging and social support. Relocation, retirement, and bereavement in later life can be considered statistically and temporally normative changes within a predictable age range (Schulz & Rau, 1985); all entail losses. The inevitability of exits from the social network, strains experienced by familial caretakers of the elderly, increased dependency, and accompanying decreased potential for reciprocity in helping exchanges have been the subject of considerable interest in the social-psychological literature.

Five nursing studies focused on this maturational change that not only potentially alters the size of the social network through loss of family and friends but also imposes strains on the existing network. The social support needs and/or resources of the elderly interested Fuller and Larson (1980), Hubbard et al. (1984), Laschinger (1984), Pohl and Fuller (1980), Powers (1985), and Brock and O'Sullivan (1985); the last three studies focused on elderly persons relocated by institutionalization. Since 1987, Beatty-Nelson's (1989) correlational, cross-sectional study of 26 institutionalized elderly persons revealed that social support was moderately correlated with self-esteem and significantly related to level of depression (see Table 5.1F).

Network Loss or Deterioration Due to Death or Divorce

The social support deficits and resources experienced by the widowed were studied by Vachon et al. (1980, 1982) and O'Brien (1985), those characteristic of single parents were examined by Norbeck and Sheiner (1982), and those evident in survivors of a volcanic eruption were analyzed by Murphy (1987). These groups consist of individuals who have experienced recent significant losses of sources of emotional, appraisal, informational, and instrumental support. These target populations also have been the foci of study in the social-psychological literature. Stroebe and Stroebe (1983) revealed that the death of a spouse leads to more negative health consequences for men than for women. Yet only one nurse researcher (O'Brien, 1985) has considered the social support needs of widowers. Since 1987, the types and primary sources of support received by 72 divorced women who had custody of 1 or more children were explored in a qualitative study that used a semistructured telephone interview (Duffy, 1989). Other women typically were identified as primary supports (see Table 5.1G).

Health Behavior and Promotion: Normal Populations

Preventive health behavior has been empirically examined by three nurse researchers in studies of residents of an adult apartment (Muhlenkamp & Sayles, 1986), women's practice of breast self-examination (Rutledge, 1987) and female employees of a large insurance company (Giersweski, 1983). Berkman (1985) postulates that lay networks exert peer pressure on health behavior and lifestyle-related activities.

Since 1987, nine studies dealt with issues of health promotion or health behavior (see Table 5.1H). Boyle's (1989) ethnographic study found that social support from a variety of sources enabled nutrition and weight control, exercise and physical fitness, and stress management in a Salvadoran population. Social support was also found to buffer anxiety for pregnant women (Norbeck & Anderson, 1989a) and had a main inverse effect on depression in a sample of adolescents (Jacobson, 1990). However, social support did not have a significant effect on self-efficacy or frequency of breast self-examination among low-income Mexican-American women (Gonzalez, 1990) or among a sample of upper-middle-class women (Rutledge, 1987). Aaronson (1989) and Albrecht and Rankin (1989) linked social support to positive health behaviors (e.g., smoking cessation, decreased alcohol consumption) among pregnant women. Two other studies discovered that health-promoting behavior and positive health status were associated with social support for elderly persons (Riffle, Yoho, & Sams, 1989; Schank & Long, 1989).

Eight studies were cross-sectional and one was longitudinal. Two were qualitative in design, using an interview schedule with a section on support. Four investigations were correlational, three were descriptive, and two were correlational-descriptive. Regrettably, none was based on a theoretical framework. Four used the same established instrument (i.e., PRQ) to measure support, and two used the NSSQ (Jacobson, 1990; Rutledge, 1987), whereas the remainder developed questions concerning sources and types of support (Boyle, 1989; Gonzalez, 1990) or participation in social and community activities (Schank & Long, 1989). Self-efficacy (Gonzalez, 1990) and self-actualization (Riffle et al., 1989) emerged as relevant variables in health behavior.

Nurses: Occupational Support

Fifteen nursing studies have examined occupational support for nurses working in a variety of sites and roles: critical care (Bizek & Oermann, 1990; Lindsey & Attridge, 1989; Norbeck, 1985d), psychiatric nurses (Cronin-Stubbs & Brophy, 1985; Cronin-Stubbs & Rooks, 1985; Hopkins-Kavanagh, 1989), public health directors (Haberman-Cohen, 1990), head nurses (Jennings, 1990), medical-surgical nurses (Ogus, 1990), nurse educators (Fong, 1990), newly employed nurses (Comi-McCloskey, 1990), nurses in a correctional setting (Skiles & Hinson, 1989), and nursing students (Marshall, 1989; Pagana, 1990) (see Table 5.1I).

All studies were cross-sectional; four were descriptive, seven were correlational, and four were correlational-descriptive. One employed LaRocco et al.'s (1980) model of occupational support-stress, and one briefly referred to coping theory (Pagana, 1990). Eleven employed a standardized social support instrument: the NSSQ (5), Social Support Questionnaire (1), Social Integration Measure (1), Inventory of Socially Supportive Behaviors (1), People Around You Scale (2), and the Malone Social Network Inventory (1). Most used other instruments measuring hardiness, job satisfaction, burnout, or psychological symptoms, and eight also measured stress.

Weak direct effects were found by Jennings (1990) on psychological symptoms. Buffering effects of support were not found on psychological symptoms (Jennings, 1990) or on burnout (Ogus, 1990; Skiles & Hinson, 1989) but were found on autonomy (McCloskey, 1990). The positive impact of support on evaluation of challenge, level of job satisfaction, health, psychological symptoms, and work performance was revealed in other studies. A more negative effect of the network was reflected in Cronin-Stubbs and Brophy's (1985) finding that frequent interpersonal contacts contributed significantly to burnout. Affect support and stability of relationships were negatively related to burnout (Cronin-Stubbs & Brophy, 1985); affirmational support was not associated with burnout (Cronin-Stubbs & Brophy, 1985). Lower amounts of positive stress and emotional support were associated with higher degrees of burnout. On- and off-job support was negatively associated with burnout; in particular, emotional support not affirmation (Cronin-Stubbs & Rooks, 1985). Norbeck (1985d) reported main but not buffering effects of social support. Work support for married nurses explained 24% of variance in perceived job stress; support from relatives explained 10% of variance in job stress and 16% of variance in psychological symptoms.

Summary and Critique

Results of Research

The main and direct effects of support and other pertinent outcomes are detailed in the last 3 columns of Table 5.1. Predominantly positive outcomes and associations are revealed. Thus social support has a positive impact by being associated with increased coping effectiveness, family functioning, physical and psychological health status, maternal attachment, self-esteem, adjustment, autonomy, adaptation, parent-infant interaction, duration of lactation, stress management, health-promoting behavior, and job satisfaction. Support also has positive outcomes in its relationship with decreased anxiety, burnout (lay and professional caregivers), psychological distress, uncertainty, and depression in a variety of populations.

Only four studies that tested the impact of social support did not find any effects of support on the variables of interest (e.g., Gonzales, 1990; Printz-Fedderson, 1990; Rutledge, 1987; Skiles & Hinson, 1989). Rarely were negative outcomes reported. One study found a negative direct effect on emotion-focused coping but a positive effect on problem-focused copers (McNett, 1987). Some would contend, however, that problem-focused coping is more effective. High social support among pregnant women was associated with substance abuse by reinforcing negative health practices (Norbeck & Anderson, 1989b). Likewise, pregnant women who lived with a smoker perceived less general support and less specific support for not smoking (Aaronson, 1989). Cronin-Stubbs & Brophy (1985) report that frequent interpersonal contacts positively contributed to burnout. The negative results of these three studies illustrate the potentially detrimental impact of interactions, due to social comparison and conflict and negative influence of some network members.

General Design Issues

Most nursing studies of social support perceived or received by different populations have been cross-sectional, quantitative, and correlational or descriptive.

Timing. Prospective studies observe a representative group on at least two occasions, following the sample for a designated period of time. Measures are employed from the present to some point in the future. Nonexperimental prospective studies start with presumed cause(s) and proceed forward in time to the presumed effect. The temporal sequences create a stronger design (Polit & Hungler, 1991; Woods & Catanzaro, 1988). Longitudinal studies are necessary to reflect and measure slowly changing processes and to characterize the course of phenomena. They are designed to observe change over time, whereas cross-sectional designs involve selecting a representative sample from populations of interest and observing phenomena at the same point in time (Woods & Catanzaro, 1988).

Qualitative or Quantitative. In the ongoing debate over qualitative versus quantitative approaches, there is growing acknowledgment that both are needed (Polit & Hungler, 1991). Some would argue, however, that these are incompatible paradigms. Quantitative research reflects the positivist school of thought, which values objective knowledge, logical inquiry and research procedures, and mechanistic and social order. In contrast, the phenomenological perspective assumes a fundamental difference between natural/physical and psychosocial sciences and emphasizes the whole person, the historical and subjective aspects of human experience, and subjects' definitions of reality (Woods & Catanzaro, 1988). The philosophy of science on which qualitative research is based is symbolic interactionism (Blumer, 1969). Research is conducted in natural settings and reality emerges as people define it.

Quantitative research is strong in generalizability, precision of information, control over extraneous variables, reliability of measures, and analytical procedures. It is useful for establishing cause-and-effect relationships, for rigorously testing research questions, and for determining the opinions, practices, and attitudes of large populations. However, validity may be problematic, as the full context of the situation and complex human experiences may be treated superficially and tightly structured questions may be biased (Polit & Hungler, 1991).

Qualitative research is useful for exploring and description, illustrating quantitative findings, discovery and exploration, and extension of theory. Data may be gathered through unstructured methods (e.g., diaries, case studies, observations, or interviewing). Data collection and analysis are designed to yield complex explanations about the natural life of persons and groups. Qualitative research is used when little is known about people, institutions, or social phenomena and if no explicit or a prior hypothesis exists. Its advantages include its flexibility, and its potential to yield in-depth insights into complex phenomena. However, the typically small and unrepresentive samples may negatively influence reliability and generalizability, and the vast amount of narrative data may be difficult to analyze (Polit & Hungler, 1991; Wilson, 1985).

"Neither of the two styles of research can fully deliver its promise to establish the truth about phenomena of interest" (Polit & Hungler, 1991). Therefore triangulation may blend different collection methods to obtain different data, check accounts for consistency (Wilson, 1985), and enrich areas of inquiry. Combination of methodologies can yield complementarity, enhance theoretical insights, enhance validity, scrutinize discrepancies, discover new frontiers, and lend insight into the multidimensionality of human phenomena.

Populations

The nursing empirical literature to date has emphasized client target populations central to the profession's activities and concerns, constituting expectant and new parents, caretakers of the ill or elderly, and the physically ill who have undergone surgery or have chronic ailments. Clearly the last group represents one significant, relevant, and valid nursing contribution to the social support literature, which does not typically address the social support concerns and resources of those with specific illnesses and disabilities. Widows, single parents, survivors of a natural disaster, and the victims of rape or abuse have been the subjects of only one or two studies each. These target groups have for the most part suffered from distress associated with deficit situations or transitions rather than acute situational stressors. (Norbeck's [1988a] review identifies nursing studies in the areas of life transitions, role performance, health behavior, and crisis or illness behavior.)

However, in considering potential target populations for future studies, researchers should address the gaps identified in the categories of age, sex, ethnic or economic context, and life-change events. To summarize, these empirical studies have overlooked children, males only, native peoples, the poor, the unemployed, the gainfully employed, and victims of child abuse or elder abuse. Nurses practice in diverse institutional and community-based sites, and hence have direct contact with all these population groups.

Children are one high-priority population that nurses should attend to initially. It is unfortunate that there is no mention in the nursing empirical literature of children's perceptions of support. Bryant (1985) clearly demonstrates that children as young as 7 years old can be reliably interviewed and that informal support sources are related to social-emotional functioning during middle childhood. This direct examination of children's social networks rather than the traditional, indirect focus on the parents' social network (e.g., Cochran & Brassard, 1979) is extremely useful because reciprocal exchanges and prosocial empathy skills must be developed in childhood. Children of separated and divorced parents have been neglected in the empirical nursing literature. They can encounter "conflicted" relations between parents and with siblings and depletion of their peer network, in addition to "loss" of a parent (e.g., Gottlieb, 1985c). Minkler (1985) claims that the elderly who are isolated or institutionalized may be disadvantaged in terms of health. Yet none of the nursing studies focuses on the social support concerns of the elderly living alone.

Only five nursing empirical studies examine relevant cultural factors, specifically, the social support needs and resources of Taiwanese patients with cancer (Lindsey et al., 1985), of African-American hysterectomized women (Jackson, 1985), and of Anglo-Latino families of children with cancer (Friedman, 1985); the health promotion factors of low-income Mexican-American women (Gonzalez, 1990) and of men and women from an urban community in El Salvador (Boyle,

1989) also were examined. Yet Vaux and Harrison (1985) claim that culture determines the extent, composition, and content of social relationships, and social support varies across subgroups of the population. Furthermore, those in lower socioeconomic groups requir particular attention (Thoits, 1983) yet, with few exceptions, receive little in the nursing social-support studies (Hall, Schaefer, & Greenberg, 1987; Norbeck & Anderson, 1989a, 1989b). Although nurses have extensively studied their own occupational stressors and support, no investigators examine support for other workers, despite the fact that occupational health nurses have early access to the recently unemployed and to employees in stressful work environments. There is recognition in the proceedings of two nursing-research conferences of the significance of cultural and socioeconomic variables (e.g., Norbeck, 1985a; Norbeck & Tilden, 1988; Tilden, 1985c) for future social support investigations.

Broader theoretical frameworks, germane to populations studied, also could enhance potential contributions to the field. The general role of theoretical frameworks as a foundation for research is delineated later in this chapter. For example, loneliness theory (Lopata, Jeinmann, & Baum, 1982; Rook, 1984; Weiss, 1974) is pertinent to studies of widows, single parents, caregivers, elderly, and the physically disabled, and social comparison theory (Shinn et al., 1984; Taylor, 1983) could explain reactions of the ill and new parents. Norbeck (1988b) astutely advises that it is time to "shift research agendas and to ask what are the key ingredients of social support that are protective for a particular population." Once this is determined, pertinent interventions can be tested by nurse investigators.

Intervention Studies

Most nursing studies have simply examined the social support currently existing in the natural environment that the respondent has actually received or perceives as a potential resource. However, professionals in empirical studies in the nursing literature reviewed prior to 1987 (Norbeck, 1988b; Stewart, 1989d) had, with five notable exceptions, not intervened to facilitate, enhance, or mobilize the informal networks of members of the target populations.

Vachon et al. (1980) detail a longitudinal, randomized control trial in which 68 of 162 widows received emotional, informational, and instrumental support from other widows, initially through one-to-one support and later in small-group sessions. The treatment group adapted to bereavement more quickly than the control group. Cronenwett (1985a) investigated changes in men's and women's relationships with social-network members from the 3rd trimester of pregnancy to 9 months postpartum. There is a very brief reference in this article to a nursing intervention, which is not detailed in any of her publications (Cronenwett, 1980, 1985b) relevant to this project. Cronenwett (1985a, p. 349) simply states that the intervention supported the most active role for the father and "facilitated" the exchange of support among couples at the same stage of family development. Doyle and Straub (1985) reported a controlled clinical trial designed to test the efficacy of an intervention by family nurse practitioners with high-risk adult populations. The intervention included one-to-one individualized sessions with various education and counseling techniques (e.g., support, guidance). and groups that were conceptualized as educational rather than as support. There were no differences between groups in perceived social support, life changes, and functional status, but intervention recipients had lower morbidity in the first 6 months. Although these are individual and group-level interventions, they seem to focus indirectly rather than directly on social support and do not involve the natural network. The focus appears to be social skills training, although this is not clear. Dracup (1985) examined the effects of spousal participation in a cardiac rehabilitation program (Dracup et al., 1985) . Both counseling-intervention groups were more effective than no group (control). Dracup suggests that support interventions should be linked to spouses separately from patients. These controlled studies include dyadic and group-level intervention by nurses but do not clearly delineate the nursing role, and there is no evidence that the authors considered other possible levels of intervention.

Since 1987, five studies have examined members of existing support or self-help groups for parents of children with chronic conditions (Betz et al., 1990), head injury victims (Hermansen-Williams, 1990), stroke survivors and their caregivers (Printz-Fedderson, 1990), persons with ostomy (Rheume & Gooding, 1991), and family members of persons in ICU (Sabo, Kraay, & Rudy, 1989) (see Table 5.2). These were all cross-sectional, qualitative, descriptive studies, not based on

(text continued on page 132)

Table 5.2 Intervention studies in nursing literature on social support since 1987

Study	*Sample*	*Design*	*Theoretical Framework*	*Stress Measure*	*Support Measure*	*Other Variables*	*Intervention*	*Outcome*
Betz et al. (1990)	32 self-help groups for parents of children with chronic conditions	Cross-sectional, descriptive, qualitative, telephone interview	—	—	Questions related to structure and function of self-help groups	—	Telephone interviews were conducted by nurses with founders or leaders of self-help groups	Function of groups are multifaceted; the majority are concerned with providing emotional support and information
Halm (1990)	25 adult family caregivers involved in support groups, 30 adult family caregivers involved in conventional bedside support	Longitudinal, quasi-experimental design, quantitative	—	—	—	State-Trait Anxiety Inventory	One 90-minute support group session involving information on nursing care, coping mechanisms, and seeking support—nurse facilitator	Group interventions can offer temporary improvement in the psychological state/anxiety of family members and help develop support networks for future coping
Hermansen-Williams (1990)	77 members of existing head-injury support groups (convenience sample)	Cross-sectional, descriptive	—	—	21 questions designed for this study assessing the impact, benefits, and description of the support group	—	Individuals were surveyed concerning the impact, benefits, and description of their membership in a head-injury support group	The support groups were beneficial for obtaining information, sharing experiences, increasing awareness and learning about resources, and increased ability to cope
Hodnett & Osborn (1989a)	103 women randomized to receive routine nursing care or routine plus one-to-one support by a monitrice	Longitudinal, qualitative, RCT	—	—	Describe differences in support 2-4 weeks postpartum	1. Labor Agentry Scale 2. Support questionnaire indicating labor support and who provided it 3. State-Trait Anxiety Inventory	Women received either routine nursing care or routine care plus one-to-one support by an experienced monitrice (support—physical comfort, emotional, advocacy)	Professional intrapartum support exerts significant direct effects on stress; support enabled labor longer at home; fewer stirrups and more intact peritoneums, less medication

Hodnett & Osborn (1989b)	103 low-risk pregnant women attending one of two prenatal education programs (traditional vs. one-to-one professional support)	Longitudinal, qualitative, RCT	—	—	—	1. State-Trait Anxiety Inventory 2. Labor Agentry Scale 3. Commitment to Unmedicated Birth, 2 items	Participants were enrolled in one of two prenatal education programs: additional prenatal and postpartum support or prenatal support and continuous intrapartum support by a familiar professional caregiver	Predictors of perceived control were expectations of control, presence of continuous professional caregiver, and pain medication usage; fewer medications and episiotomies in experimental group
Jessop & Stein (1991)	174 children with a variety of chronic conditions	Longitudinal, qualitative-quantitative	—	—	—	1. Judged ability to cope 2. Clinician's Overall Burden Index 3. Satisfaction with Care Schedule 4. Psychiatric Symptom Index	Professional pedi-atric home care program (interdisciplinary) provides integrated medical and psychosocial services	Maximal benefit evident when illness burden was small but coping resources (e.g., social, educational) were low; social factors most important, not medical
Killien & Shy (1989)	135 women assigned to electronic fetal monitoring or periodic consultation for preterm labor	Cross-sectional (randomized clinical trial)	—	Indicators of potential stress: birth weight, 1- and 5-minutes Apgar scores, and gestational age	Intrapartum care: perceptions of medical and nursing support (49 items)	1. Preparation for labor, personal and infant characteristics, knowledge and expectations of monitoring, and prenatal class attendance 2. Global measure evaluating labor 3. Perceived control-modification of labor evaluation scale	Examined the perceptions of preterm labor and birth for women who experienced electronic fetal monitoring or periodic auscultation; all cared for by one-to-one study nurses	Women's evaluation of the labor event was strongly influenced by perceptions of nursing support, not technological intervention; no significant differences on any other study measures

(*Continued*)

Table 5.2 (Continued)

Study	*Sample*	*Design*	*Theoretical Framework*	*Stress Measure*	*Support Measure*	*Other Variables*	*Intervention*	*Outcome*
McCullough et al. (1989)	40 patients who experienced temporal lobectomy for seizure control engaged in a follow-up program	Longitudinal, qualitative, descriptive	—	—	Interview questions concerning post-operative social changes	Interview designed by investigators assessing physical, emotional, and cognitive post-operative changes	Follow-up multidisciplinary program for patients who experienced anterior temporal lobectomy involving psychosocial support and information (reassurance, information, bolster self-esteem, and coping mechanisms)	For families with poor family support, regular contact with follow-up staff or peer groups was important for feedback and assurance (speculate enable recovery process)
Mohide et al. (1990)	60 caregivers of older people suffering from moderate to severe progressive irreversible dementia and caregivers suffering from depression and anxiety	Longitudinal, quantitative, descriptive, RCT	—	—	Descriptive data on support service utilization, health, and caregiving	1. Center for Epidemiologic Studies Depression Scale 2. State-Trait Anxiety Inventory 3. Caregiver Quality of Life Index 4. Time Trade-Off Technique 5. Cantril Self-Anchoring Striving Scale 6. Interview—service needs	Experimental intervention: caregiver-focused health care, education about dementia and caregiving, assistance with problem solving, regular in-home respite, and a self-help caregiver support group; control group: conventional community nursing care (6-month intervention)	No significant differences for depression or anxiety; the intervention group showed improvement in quality of life, a longer mean time to long-term institutionalization, fewer problems with caregiving, and greater satisfaction with nursing care than did controls
Montgomery-Hunter & Striden-Hall (1989)	8 adults participating in an existing support group for individuals with COPD	Longitudinal, qualitative, descriptive	—	—	—	1. Profile of Mood States 2. Questionnaire on dyspnea developed by researchers 3. Educational material distributed on COPD	Support group involving an educational and small-group discussion component for 2 hours a week for 5 weeks for patients with COPD	Subjects expressed that the program helped in coping even though the support and educational program did not decrease exacerbations of dyspnea or improve emotional status (scores on Profile of Mood States)

Printz-Fedderson (1990)	40 stroke survivors with known caregivers and 40 caregivers with known stroke club involvement	Expost facto design, qualitative, descriptive, not randomized	—	—	—	1. Physical Caregiving Responsibility Inventory 2. The Geriatric Depression Scale 3. CADET (physical burden)	Caregivers were assessed who had attended one stroke club event within the previous 6 months; the primary service of the support group was a source of friendship, emotional support, education, and information	Support group members reported low levels of depression and perceived burden but not significant
Rheume & Gooding (1991)	26 adults recruited from 2 united ostomy groups	Cross-sectional, qualitative, descriptive	—	—	Personal Resource Questionnaire	1. Jalowiec Coping Scale 2. Quality of Life Index	Participants were involved in existing group meetings on a monthly basis to discuss physical and psychosocial issues of ostomy management	High levels of perceived support, more problem-focused coping than affective coping, and high scores on quality of life and low scores on physical well-being
Sabo et al. (1989)	31 family members who attended an ICU support group session, 36 controls	Cross-sectional, qualitative, descriptive	—	10 questions assessing feelings of stress (based on Lazarus, 1981)	9 questions assessing feelings of social support (adapted from PRQ)	Questions assessing perceived benefits of attending a support group and feelings of hope	ICU family support group session; no descriptions provided	Attending an ICU support group did not significantly change stress, hope, or social support
Thompson (1989)	60 male patients with first myocardial infarction and their partners (30 treatment and 30 control)	Longitudinal, quantitative, qualitative, RCT	—	—	—	1. Coronary Prognostic Index 2. Hospital Anxiety and Depression Scale 3. Health data: heart rate, blood pressure, and body mass index	Intervention consisted of a systemic supportive-educational counseling program of nursing support in addition to routine care; the control group received routine care	Average scores for patient anxiety and depression were decreased in comparison to the control group; no effect for partner anxiety or depression

a theoretical framework. Although Printz-Fedderson employed an ex post facto comparison design, no intervention was applied and subjects were not randomly allocated. Printz-Fedderson (1990) and Rheume and Gooding (1991) both administered structured scales and instruments; however, only the latter used a social support scale. Benefits of support-group membership were described in terms of increased information, lower levels of depression and perceived burden, more problem-focused coping, and higher quality of life.

Nine "intervention" studies have been conducted with family caregivers (Halm, 1990; Mohide et al., 1990; Sabo et al., 1989), pregnant women (Hodnett & Osborn, 1989a, 1989b; Killien & Shy, 1989), new mothers (Elliot, Sanjack, & Leverton, 1988), individuals with COPD (Montgomery-Hunter & Striden-Hall, 1989), persons with their first myocardial infarction (MI) and their partners (Thompson, 1989), children with chronic illness (Jessop & Stein, 1991), and persons who had undergone temporal lobectomy for seizure control (McCullough, Day, Herlihy, & Rapp, 1989) (Table 5.2). Five of these interventions, although support-oriented, actually encompassed professional support only, whether by nurses (Thompson, 1989) or others (Hodnett & Osborn, 1989a; Jessop & Stein, 1991; Killien & Shy, 1989; McCullough et al., 1989). All five studies were longitudinal; one was qualitative, one was quantitative, and two were combined quantitative-qualitative. Support in these professional support studies was associated with decreased anxiety, depression, and medication use and with increased perceived control.

One intervention entailed one-to-one support by an experienced monitrice (lay midwife) (Hodnett & Osborn, 1989b). Only two studies involved support or support-educational group interventions (i.e., Halm, 1990; Montgomery-Hunter & Striden-Hall, 1989). Mohide et al. (1990) combined a support group for caregivers of seniors with dementia not only with education but also with in-home respite. Thus only four studies actually entailed lay support interventions; only two of these used a true randomized control trial design (Halm, 1990; Hodnett & Osborn, 1989b). All four were longitudinal (Table 5.2).

Elliot et al. (1988) conducted a controlled trial using parent groups as a preventive intervention for postnatal depression. The investigators (one a nurse midwife) recognized the importance of social comparison offering groups of "similar others." The focus was educational; early sessions were more structured, and open discussion time increased in later sessions. A small pilot test provided information on optimum numbers of members and timing and structuring of meetings. The program was successful in reducing the prevalence of depression in new mothers only. Halm (1990) describes the effects of support groups on reducing family members' anxiety during critical times. The control group received conventional support by professionals in the hospital, whereas the experimental group benefited from additional group sessions, facilitated by a nurse, by sharing feelings and experiences in coping with critical illness. These were 90-minute sessions that focused on coping mechanisms, care, and seeking support. Group interventions offered temporary improvement in psychological state and helped the family to develop support networks for future coping.

The lay support interventions were found to improve quality of life, delay institutionalization, diminish problems with caregiving (Mohide et al., 1990), diminish anxiety (Halm, 1990; Hodnett and Osborn, 1989b), and increase hope (not measured) (Montgomery-Hunter & Striden-Hall, 1989). A direct effect on stress and anxiety was revealed in Hodnett & Osborn's (1989b) intervention. However, the support intervention in Montgomery-Hunter and Striden-Hall's study did not decrease dyspnea or improve emotional status in COPD patients.

Critique

The gaps identified above point to the need for intervention studies conducted by nurse investigators. Schmitt (1985), summarizing the themes of a symposium for nurse researchers interested in social support, observed that "most of the symposium was devoted to papers that one might call more basic than applied—there were relatively few research reports of intervention studies" (p. 231). Cohen and Syme (1985), among others, recognize this gap in social-psychological and medical publications. Hence it should be acknowledged that the unfortunate rarity of intervention studies is not limited to the nursing contributions to social support literature. Recent books published by Vaux (1989) and Gottlieb (1988a) overcame this deficit to some extent.

The virtual absence of empirical studies about social support interventions may reflect a more deep-seated omission in the practice of professional nurses. Nurses should overcome institutional barriers and avoid ostracism of the natural-network members. On the other hand, nurses may do many of the support-enhancing behaviors now, but they are not being studied or evaluated in any systemic way. We need to affirm their actions and support efforts to evaluate these behaviors (Brink, 1987). Furthermore, as Norbeck (1985a) suggests, "The large and ponderous question of how social support works will have to be addressed before sound intervention programs can be designed" (p. 12).

Social support "came of age" as a complex phenomenon of interest and significance in mainline social-behavioral health research only in the past decade. It takes time to do the preliminary exploratory, descriptive, and correlational studies that underpin later intervention studies (Brink, 1987). Furthermore, by the time research is completed and appears in print, a significant amount of time has elapsed. These may be reasons that more intervention studies have not yet appeared in the literature. Although intervention studies are undoubtedly important, Rook and Dooley's (1985) cautionary comment should be considered: "Social support achieved through interventions should not be assumed to be equivalent in its form or effects to social support normally available from one's family and friends" (p. 10). Thus, although there is clearly a consultative and facilitative role for nurses and other professionals with respect to natural and created network sources of social support, the "artificial" connotations of such support could be considered problematic. On the other hand, this may be a positive feature in cases where "support" available from the natural network is inadequate, nonexistent, or fraught with conflict and strain.

Intervention strategies, proposed in Chapter 4 and described in this section, can be implemented in longitudinal studies to see whether gains are maintained (Gottlieb, 1988a). Longitudinal designs permit prospective analyses and examination of the level of social support over time (Cutrona, Russell, & Rose, 1986) and unanticipated side effects, concurrent losses, and "unplanned" lay interventions (Gottlieb, 1988b). Observations of process and outcome of individual, dyadic, and group-level interventions could be recorded. Outcomes were exemplified in Chapter 4, and satisfaction with quality as well as quantity of potential and actual social support and social network should be elicited from both recipients and providers in treatment groups and control groups.

Controlled intervention trials are needed to test interventions (Norbeck, 1988b) based on theory. There is a continuum of design types in terms of capacity to reveal causal relationships, moving from true experimental to quasi-experimental to path analytic to prospective correlational to retrospective correlation (Polit & Hungler, 1991). Basic research or pure research provides the building blocks for increments in knowledge and further research. In contrast, applied or intervention research includes studies directed to solving practical problems and making clinical decisions, as well as clinical trials aimed at developing and evaluating new programs, products, methods, and procedures (Wilson, 1985). Some researchers have successfully used true-experimental designs in evaluating support programs, but most rely on quasi-experimental designs with their attendant problems. An untreated control or comparison group to which participants are assigned randomly is desirable. The use of interventions with multiple components can pose problems in discovering potent elements (Vaux, 1989). Nurses, through easy direct contact with clientele and their networks in health-care facilities and community-based sites, are particularly familiar with diverse populations. Empirical intervention research conducted by appropriately educated nurses should enhance future practical and theoretical development of the social support field.

Measures of Social Support

Twenty-six measuring instruments developed by nurse researchers were reviewed (Stewart, 1989c). Only one third of the measures include reported results of reliability and validity testing. In several cases, the authors expressed justifiable concerns with the results. Norbeck's (1988a) review of 67 nurse-authored research articles reveals that only 28% of 40 studies in which social support was directly measured as a study variable used instruments with established reliability and validity. Perhaps repeated application of a few instruments to different target populations is needed to establish reliability.

In this context, only three instruments have undergone significant psychometric testing (see Table 5.3). The Tilden Interpersonal Relationship Inventory (IPRI) (1988) evolved from the Tilden (1985a) Cost and Reciprocity of Social Support scale (CARSS). The latter was revised and reformulated through repeated administration to small samples and pilot tested on 28 normal persons. Tilden and Galyen (1987) and Tilden, Nelson, and May (1990) describe how, during its initial development, 44 adults in the community experiencing a range of life situations were interviewed to develop 140 items indexing

(text continued on page 139)

Table 5.3 Reliability and Validity for CARSS/IPRI, NSSQ, and PRQ

			Reliability		*Validity*		
Instrument	*Study*	*Sample*	*Internal Consistency*	*Test/Retest*	*Content*	*Construct*	*Criterion*
IPRI	Tilden (1988)	235 subjects: students, cancer patients, adult women, patients in an obesity program, and hypercholestermia patients.	—	—	—	Tested with a stress measure, second social support measure, and measure of social desirability; all variables had main or interaction effects except reciprocity	Moderate to high correlations between subscales and support subscale of FRI, and moderate correlation between IPRI and PRQ
	Tilden, Nelson, & May (1990)	44 adults experiencing a range of life situations (cancer, homelessness)	—	—	Panel of 11 judges reduced 140 items to 74 (interrater reliability 92.3%)	—	—
		43 undergraduate nurses	Support .92 Reciprocity .83 Conflict .91	Support .91 Reciprocity .84 Conflict .81	Reduced to 39 items	—	—
NSSQ	Norbeck et al. (1983)	136 staff employees at a large university medical center	—	—	—	Administered the Fundamental Interpersonal Relations Orientation (FIRO-B) Questionnaire; two constructs of the FIRO-B (need for inclusion and need for affection) were related to all social support functional scales (.18 to .27) and to the network scales (.17 to .23); correlations with need for control were not significant as predicted	—

NSSQ	Norbeck et al. (1983)	55 female graduate nursing students	—	—	—	—	Tested concurrent validity with PRQ and predictive validity in relation to the stress buffering role of social support (LES and POMS); significant associations between NSSQ and PRQ (.35 to .41) and lower levels for the network properties (.31 to .32)
	Norbeck (1984)	75 graduate nursing students	Affect .97 Affirmation .96 Aid .89	Functional and network properties ranged from .85 to .92	—	—	—
		42 graduate nursing students	—	—	—	—	Tested concurrent validity with the SSQ; affirmation and informational support (.33), affect and emotional support (.51), but aid was not related to SSQ measure of tangible support
PRQ82	Weinert (1983)	181 adults responded to open-ended questions	—	—	Two judges (nurse researchers) and one content specialist determined 8 domains from 123 responses (part 1)	Correlated perceived social support scale with scores on the Beck Depression Inventory and the Trait Anxiety Scale; significant moderate correlations between PRQ82—Part 2 and BDI ($r = -.33$) and the Trait Anxiety Scale ($r = -.39$)	—
		120 adults responded to open-ended questions	—	—	Two judges (nurse researchers) and one content specialist determined 8 domains from 112 responses (part 1)	—	—

(Continued)

Table 5.3 (Continued)

			Reliability		Validity		
Instrument	*Study*	*Sample*	*Internal Consistency*	*Test/Retest*	*Content*	*Construct*	*Criterion*
PRQ85	Muhlenkamp (1985)	132 older persons living in trailer parks or mobile-home settings	Total scale .87 Nurturance subscale (Cronbach's alpha) .62	—	—	—	—
	Catanzaro (1986)	100 middle-aged adults	Total scale .90 Nurturance subscale .68	—	—	—	—
	Weinert (1987)	132 middle-aged adults	Total scale .89 Nurturance subscale .64	—	—	—	—
	Weinert & Tilden (1990)	333 middle-aged adults	Total scale .90	—	—	—	—
		99 adults (white, urban, middle class)	Total scale .91	—	—	Profile of Mood States used to assess association between social support and indices of negative mood states (-.31)	—
PRQ85 Part 2	Higgins & Dicharry (1991)	29 Navajo women	—	—	10 items of the total 25 culturally unacceptable (80% level of acceptance required)	—	—

interpersonal support, reciprocity, and conflict, which were reduced to 74 items during content-validity assessment and later to 39 items following testing on a sample of students. The Cost and Reciprocity Index (CRI), which yields scores for social support, reciprocity, cost, and conflict, was then tested on 2 samples. Cost, however, was not a strong factor (Kirschling, Tilden, & Butterfield, 1990). Construct-validity testing with 235 subjects revealed that all variables had main or interaction effects except reciprocity, which correlated highly with social support (Tilden, 1988). Criterion validity was measured with the Norbeck Social Support Questionnaire (NSSQ), Inventory of Socially Supportive Behaviors (ISSB), Interpersonal Support Evaluation List (ISEL), Profile of Mood States, and Social Support Scales (Weinert & Tilden, 1990).

The NSSQ, based on Kahn's definition of support, measures affect, affirmation and aid, network properties, and recent losses (Norbeck, 1988a). It was tested on a sample of 75 graduate nursing students and 642 senior nursing students. High levels of test-retest reliability and internal consistency were reported and moderate levels of concurrent validity were found (Norbeck, 1984). By 1983, a small normative base was established and predictive validity was found in a sample of 55 graduate students reflecting the stress-buffering role hypothesized for social support. Studies found that the instrument was free from social-desirability response bias, stable over a 7-month period, and sensitive to changes in networks. Construct validity with another social support questionnaire, the PRQ, was found (Norbeck et al., 1983). Concurrent validity was tested with PRQ and the Social Support Questionnaire, and predictive validity was tested (detailed in Norbeck, 1984). This instrument has been used in numerous studies by other authors (see Table 5.1).

The Personal Resources Questionnaire (PRQ) is a self-administered questionnaire; Part 1 measures situational support and Part 2 is a global measure of perceived social support. The PRQ, Part 1, lists 8 life situations representing domains of events when a person might need assistance. Content validity was initially established with a team of experts adding a 9th question, and with another two samples necessitating 2 additional questions. Five dimensions of social support are measured: intimacy, social integration, nurturance, worth, and assistance. Factor analysis revealed 3 factors: Intimacy/Assistance, Integration/Affirmation, and Reciprocity. Psychometric testing revealed strong internal consistency. The PRQ 85 has moderate negative correlations with mood states and higher correlations with measures of family well-being and other theoretically relevant variables than the CRI (Weinert & Tilden, 1990). Moderate intercorrelations among subscales were found consistently. Higgins and Dicharry (1991) assessed content validity of the PRQ, Part 2, with 29 Navajo women. Ten items were considered to be culturally unacceptable (e.g., discuss personal feelings, family problems). Items considered acceptable concerned belonging to a group, nurturant behavior, and emotional help.

The PRQ (Brandt & Weinert, 1981; Weinert, 1987; Weinert & Brandt, 1987) was compared to the NSSQ by Brandt (1984b), who indicated that both were designed to measure aspects of relational and structural network dimensions. Although similar relational content is measured by both, the PRQ measures opportunity for nurturing support. Neither assesses relational dimensions of symmetry, strength, or personal interconnectedness. Size, diversity, and stability are tapped by the NSSQ, whereas only network density is measured by the PRQ (Brandt, 1984b). Weinert and Tilden (1990) contrasted the PRQ with Tilden's CRI and found that although both measure the construct of social support, they assess different aspects. However, the CRI's correlations with theoretically relevant variables tend to be lower than the PRQ.

The eight dimensions selected to form the evaluative framework used in the earlier review (Stewart, 1989c) of nursing instruments explicated source (network members providing support), disposition (availability or enactment), duration (stability of support), type (functional content or categories of properties/functions), positive or negative (benefits or drawbacks/costs of support), direction (given and/or received support), described or evaluated (features of or satisfaction with support), and level (interaction of these seven dimensions). The three tested instruments are described according to these dimensions in Table 5.4.

Critique

In sum, duration of support, mutual receipt and provision of support, costs associated with negative support, and evaluation of satisfaction with support are infrequently assessed. Further the specific level of social support is at best inconsistently measured. Finally,

Table 5.4 Instruments Developed by Nurse Researchers to Measure Social Support (SS)

Scale	*Positive/ Negative*	*Direction*	*Disposition*	*Description Evaluation*	*Type/Content*	*Source/ Network (SN)*	*Duration*	*Level*
Brandt & Weinert (1981) Personal Resource Questionnaire (Brandt, 1984a, 1984b; Higgins & Dicharry, 1991; Weinert, 1987; Weinert & Brandt, 1987)	+	Received	Enacted, available	Described, evaluated	Emotional, instrumental, appraisal	Family, (close) friends, professionals, books, prayers	Recall social support over past 6 months	25-item, 7-point Likert scale measured perceived level of SS
Norbeck et al. (1981) Social Support Questionnaire (Norbeck, 1985a, 1988a; Norbeck et al., 1983)	+	Received	Available	Described	Emotional, instrumental, appraisal	(0–12) Counselor, minister, spouse/partner, family, friends, coworkers, neighbors, professionals	"How long have you known"—less than 6 months, more than 5 years; SN losses past year	1. Likert scale, "How much does it make you feel" 2. SN size 3. Frequency
Tilden, Nelson, & May (1990) Interpersonal Relationship Inventory (Kirschling, Tilden, & Butterfield, 1990; Tilden, 1985a; Tilden & Galyen, 1987; Tilden & Stewart, 1985; Weinert & Tilden, 1990)	+ −	Received, provided	Enacted	Evaluated	Emotional, instrumental, informational, appraisal (implied not explicit)	Not specified (5 most important)	—	Likert scale satisfaction

few researchers operationalized important typologies in the social-psychological literature or explicated the connection between the theoretical framework of the study and the measure developed. Nevertheless, Tilden (1985a; Tilden & Galyen, 1987) based her instrument directly on equity and social exchange theories.

Because nurse researchers cannot take into account all of the possible elements or dimensions (e.g., direction, density, content, cost, reciprocity), they will have to select those with the highest payoff. Research designed to evaluate the actual effect from these elements will expedite identification of categories that are essential to validate the information elicited and those that are merely germane or advisable additions to instruments. As Norbeck (personal communication, 1986) recommended researchers should determine whether such elements add to the predictive power of social support in the stress-social support-health models.

O'Reilly's (1988) review of 24 social support measures and of 9 social network measures revealed the confusion resulting from including components of social networks in conceptions of social support. Subjective measures assess subjects' understanding and evaluation of support and perceptions of relationship adequacy. Objective measures quantify types of interactions, network size, and density, and usually gather information from people other than the target (Ryan & Austin, 1989). "Measures range from those with few items tapping social participation/integration to those with many items or intensive interview probing regarding sources, types, duration, mutuality and frequency of social support along with satisfaction indicators" (Gottlieb & Selby, 1989). Yet measures combining several dimensions have low reliabilities.

There are no measures of social support for ethnic or cultural groups (Gottlieb & Selby, 1989). Interview guides or instruments must be translated and tested for relevance and appropriateness (Norbeck & Tilden, 1988). Our own research with persons with hemophilia and HIV/AIDS encountered difficulty in interpreting support and coping dimensions in an interview schedule translated from English to French (Hart et al., 1991).

It is noteworthy that so many different instruments have been devised by nurses, yet only a few have been used in studies other than those in which they were first described. In this context, nurse authors of empirical studies infrequently use tested instruments included in the social-psychological literature. Perhaps the reluctance to use established instruments from other disciplines is attributable in part to the general state of dissatisfaction with the adequacy of measurement of social support and in part to a drive to create clinically relevant nursing instruments. The evidence from this review, that instruments from other disciplines are rarely applied in nursing studies, may illustrate a trend to develop measures to reflect the professional practice of nursing. However, the abundance of diverse social support measures also might be considered superfluous. The proliferation of social support measures is not limited to the nursing literature, however, as is evident in the reviews by Gottlieb and Selby (1989), House and Kahn (1985), O'Reilly (1988), Popiel and Susskind (1985), and Tardy (1985).

Norbeck (1988b) concludes that validated general instruments should be used, unless situation-specific measures are warranted. Norbeck (1985b) pointed to the promising strategy of using situation-specific measures in clinically focused social support studies and the feasibility of including situation-specific items in existing instruments. A few of the instruments developed for expectant/new parent populations do incorporate situation-specific items. Nursing contributions in this direction have been indirectly acknowledged by House and Kahn (1985), who purported that "a number of other investigators have developed and used measures of social support in small specialized non-student populations—among the most promising measures of this type are those of Norbeck et al. (1981), Brandt and Weinert (1981), and Cronenwett (1984)" (pp. 96-97). Although 26 instruments exist in reports in the nursing literature, many of them were designed to be study-specific and not of general applicability, as were the PRQ, NSSQ, CARSS, and IPRI (Interpersonal Relationships Inventory). Surely situation- and population-specific measures are a valid focus of nurse investigators' expanded efforts to develop and modify measuring instruments. This would lead not to further proliferation of instruments, but rather to enhanced relevance of existing social support instruments through supplementation.

Theory Application and Testing

Theoretical frameworks of nursing empirical studies of social support and theoretical bases of nursing instruments designed for measuring social support yield insight into the current status of the theoretical development of the social support construct by nurses.

Theoretical Frameworks of Empirical Nursing Studies of Social Support

A conceptual or theoretical framework structures the study and the research process (Brink & Wood, 1983; Wilson, 1985). These frameworks help to explain, describe, and analyze the ideas inherent in the research questions, in a logical, orderly, coherent way. They constitute the mechanism by which researchers organize empirical findings into meaningful patterns (Brink & Wood, 1983; Polit & Hungler, 1991). These frameworks or models use concepts as building blocks that have relevance to the research aims. Frameworks are the creative integration of pertinent knowledge to clarify assumptions, suggest variables and relationships, clarify the meaning of the research goal, and identify whether new knowledge is needed about how to produce desired outcomes. This sets the stage for the purposes of the study, explicates the investigator's perspective on the problem, and provides direction for the study design (Woods & Catanzaro, 1988).

Theory is basic to science and philosophy (Wilson, 1985). Theory construction and testing are intimately related to the advancement of scientific knowledge (Polit & Hungler, 1991). Theory-generating research designed to discover and describe phenomena employs inductive reasoning. Inductive reasoning moves from particular observations and facts to generalizations. A theory is developed or created inductively from observations in empirical research that validates concepts and relations (Polit & Hungler, 1991; Wilson, 1985) through grounded theory or phenomenological inquiry (Woods & Catanzaro, 1988). Deductive reasoning, which infers a particular conclusion from a set of general observations, guides theory-testing research to determine how accurately a theory accounts for observations. Theoretical relationships are translated into testable hypotheses. Hypothesis-testing studies of causal relationships contribute to explanatory and predictive theory (Polit & Hungler, 1991; Woods & Catanzaro, 1988). In short, "theory guides and generates ideas for research; research assesses the worth of the theory and provides a foundation for new ones" (Polit & Hungler, 1991, p. 117). Fawcett (1989) describes the relationship between research and theory as reciprocal—with theory as the impetus for scientific investigation and research findings shaping the development of theory. It is advantageous to place research problems into a theoretical context, either inductively or deductively. However, there is a danger in artificially fitting a problem to a theory.

A review of the theoretical frameworks of the empirical nursing studies on social support revealed that none applied social comparison, equity, loneliness, social learning, and attribution theories in their investigations. Reciprocity was inductively identified in a qualitative study of abused women (Henderson, 1989) and loneliness was alluded to by Florian and Krulik (1991). Coping theory has been invoked by four nurse investigators (Dormire et al., 1989; Lindgren, 1990; McNett, 1987; Saunders & McCorkle, 1987). Crisis theory formed the base of Halm's (1990) study of adults undergoing surgery, and depression theories underpin Jacobson's (1990) examination of normal adolescents. Three studies cited nursing theories (i.e., Orem's Self-Care Model, Kim's Collaborative Model of Decision-Making, and King's Open Systems Model) and McCubbin (1989) called upon her 1987 Typology Model of Adjustment and Adaptation. Frequently, definitions of social support are derived from pioneer authors' work. Models of occupational stress and support ground the investigations of nurses' occupational support. No intervention studies were based on theoretical frameworks.

There is a noticeable and unfortunate absence of reference to social comparison theory in the nursing literature. Certainly it is relevant to the social support associated with target groups of nursing studies, namely the bereaved, the ill, new parents, and the elderly. It is safe to assume that these people, like the cancer victims studied by Taylor (1983), would make upward comparisons with those coping better than they are, for modeling purposes, and downward comparisons to enhance self-esteem.

As observed earlier, equity theory can explain the imbalanced exchange of resources between the elderly and their caretakers. Further, the chronically ill and disabled have few opportunities to reciprocate. Yet this theory is not cited in any studies pertaining to these populations.

It is noteworthy that the nursing studies on widows (Vachon et al., 1980, 1982), single parents (Norbeck & Sheiner, 1982), and divorced women (Duffy, 1989) do not invoke loneliness theory, although it is clearly applicable to these types of losses. Loneliness theory has obvious relevance to many elderly persons living alone and in institutions. It could be incorporated by nursing authors (e.g., Beatty-

Nelson, 1989) who examine this target population. Often the physically disabled also may live alone and have limited contact outside the home. Rook (1984) maintains that loneliness arises when a person feels estranged, misunderstood, or rejected by others. Surely this applies to the chronically ill, who may suffer from social loneliness due to the restrictions of their illness. Yet these nursing studies do not cite loneliness theories, or even attribution theories, which can explain the estrangement, loneliness, and rejection resulting from reactions to the physically ill.

There is evidence that people discourage open communication and give conflicting behavioral cues in cancer patients' presence. Taylor (1983) calls upon attribution theory to interpret these reactions. Unfortunately reference to attribution theory is not incorporated in these nursing studies on social support and physical illness. Attribution theory would be a useful adjunct to Lindsey et al.'s (1985) and Clements et al.'s (1990) studies that examine the family's reaction to the cancer patient.

The virtual neglect of coping theories in the empirical literature is surprising in light of the 11 studies of chronically ill persons, 14 studies of caregivers, and 9 studies of new parents, which do not cite coping as a framework. By focusing attention on social support as a resource to facilitate coping with this stressor, coping theory could have enriched Mercer et al.'s (1984) and Richardson's (1987) research on childbirth. Use of coping theory would move these studies one step beyond the effect of support on subjective perception of childbirth, to its impact on adaptation and functioning during this experience. Finally, social learning theory could have been invoked in the 10 studies of self-help groups, to reflect role modeling inherent in such groups. Furthermore, Gonzalez (1990), Aaronson (1989), and other health promotion studies might have benefited from applying self-efficacy theory.

Theoretical Bases of Nursing Instruments

Norbeck (1985b) contends that "the conceptual linkage of social-support constructs with broader theories such as attachment, role, exchange . . . and stress and coping provide guidance for the selection of relevant components and measurement strategies" (p. 91). However, these broad theories are not explicitly acknowledged in nursing instruments with two notable exceptions. First, Tilden (1985a, 1988) derives her Cost and Reciprocity of Social Support Scale and subsequent Interpersonal Relationship Inventory directly from social exchange and equity theory. Second, Norbeck and Tilden (1983), Cranley (1984), and Zachariah (1985) based their instruments in part on attachment theory. This is appropriate in view of their target populations of expectant parents.

The lack of emphasis on reciprocity and social comparison in most nursing measures is interesting, not only in light of chronically ill and caregiver samples studied, but also in view of 10 "intervention" studies of self-help or support groups; such groups focus on mutual, reciprocal aid as a primary form of support and encompass upward and downward social comparison processes.

Attribution theory could have informed Woods and Earp's (1978) "help" subscale of their Social Support Index applied to cancer patients. According to the unique helping orientations developed by Brickman et al. (1982), responsibility for causing or solving a problem can be attributed by potential help-givers to the individual rather than the environment, leading to nonsupport and unhelpful behaviors.

Loneliness theory might have enhanced Brandt and Weinert's (1981) Personal Resource Questionnaire, which they applied to the study of multiple sclerosis victims and spousal ability to sustain family functioning. Frequently, caretakers of the chronically ill and those who are visibly disabled can be socially isolated and suffer from chronic feelings of loneliness. Therefore size of network and satisfaction with support received, measured by their instrument, could be interpreted in the context of loneliness theory.

Empirically Based Theory Development Pertinent to Social Support

Nurses have contributed to the conceptualization of social support through their research. For example, Hubbard et al. (1984) described the relationship between social support and self-care practices in a correlational study of senior citizens. Brown (1986b) empirically tested a conceptually derived multidimensional formulation of social support with a sample of expectant couples. The idea of multidimensionality was not confirmed. Brown's finding is supported by nurse researchers Norbeck (1985a) and McNett (1987). In contrast, Barrera (1986), a psychologist, purports that the global concept of social support should be abandoned in favor of more precise concepts such as social embeddedness, perceived support, and enacted support.

Since 1987, four studies have incorporated the development or testing of models (see Table 5.5). Ferketich and Mercer (1990) derived a causal model proposing that negative life events and pregnancy stress affect perceived health status indirectly, and that self-esteem, social support, relationship with mate, and family functioning have indirect effects on health status through a sense of mastery and parental competence. The model was supported with minor revisions in a longitudinal study. McNett's (1987) causal model hypothesized that perceived availability of social support, perceived effectiveness of social support, and perceived personal constraints have an impact on degree of threat and coping responses and in turn on coping effectiveness. Findings from McNett's study of functionally disabled persons revealed that perceived availability, not use of social support, was significantly and positively related to coping effectiveness, mediated by emotion- and problem-focused coping (i.e., the model fit the data). Yarcheski and Mahon (1989) developed a causal model of positive health practices for adolescents. Significant correlations were found between social support and positive health practices, and between social support and self-esteem. (The causal model was tested using path analysis via a LISREL program.) Social support had direct effects on self-esteem and on positive health practices and an indirect effect on health practices through self-esteem. In fact, social support had the strongest total effect on positive health practices of all variables. The model, however, required modification for this population. Swanson (1991) employed a phenomenological design to develop a theory of caring, which encompassed Benner's theory and Cobb's conceptualization of social support. Five caring processes that were empirically defined in her three prenatal studies were "knowing," "being with," "doing for," "enabling," and "maintaining belief."

Critique

The theoretical gap in the theoretical frameworks of social support studies in the nursing literature reemerges in the context of discussion of measuring instruments. Unfortunately, "broad" theories such as coping, attribution, loneliness, social comparison, social learning, and equity generally are overlooked. In view of Norbeck's (1988a) recommendation for theoretically based support intervention trials, it is indeed unfortunate that none of the intervention studies had theoretical frameworks. Accordingly, theoretical frameworks and measures for social support studies by nurses will have to be expanded to emphasize the multifaceted nature of social support and relevant "broad" theories.

"Conceptual work is needed to distinguish the various conditions underlying inadequate social support in order to match interventions with the appropriate need" (Norbeck, 1988b, p. 104). Cost, conflict, and stresses of support require investigation (Ryan & Austin, 1989). Researchers should consider everyday support and support at critical times (O'Reilly, 1988). Furthermore, international research is needed to test whether social support is truly a universal construct (Norbeck & Tilden, 1988).

The lack of linkage between conceptual definitions and operationalization is a prevalent deficiency (O'Reilly, 1988). Little consensus exists on how to measure social support because of the variability in definitions and conceptualizations. The construct validation of measures, however, will help develop credible social support theory (Weinert & Tilden, 1990).

Conclusion

Social support has received considerable attention by nurse investigators. "A sizeable contribution has been made by nurse researchers to understanding and quantifying the nature of social support and its relation to various facets of health and illness" (Downs, 1989, p. 133). Ethnographic approaches could, however, promote independent, intensive assessment of the dynamic process and interrelationships of support giving and receiving. Interview guides used at several points in time could include changes in costs and satisfaction with type of support for type of perceived need. Research should proceed from exploratory and descriptive research (abundant in nursing research to date) to experimental and quasi-experimental research, clinical trials, field trials (evaluation), and application to practice. Critical remaining issues for social support research by nurses, in addition to research methodologies, include the need to learn how social support works (e.g., timing, importance of specific sources, and key types for specific situations; essential characteristics of support; and gender and other individual differences), to interpret paradoxical and negative findings,

(text continued on page 152)

Table 5.5 Theory Testing in Nursing Literature on Social Support Since 1987

							Effect/Outcomes		
Study	*Sample*	*Design*	*Theoretical Framework*	*Stress Measure*	*Support Measure*	*Other Measures*	*Main*	*Buffering*	*Results*
Ferketich & Mercer (1990)	87 high-risk-pregnancy women and 139 low-risk-pregnancy women	Cross-sectional, correlational, quantitive	Causal model involving self-esteem, social support, and health status	1. Negative Life Events Survey 2. Pregnancy Risk Score 3. Intrapartal Risk Score	1. Inventory of Socially Supportive Behaviors 2. Checklist of Supportive Persons, 6 items on perceived support	1. General Health Index 2. Self-Esteem Scale 3. Sense of Mastery 4. Parental Sense of Competence 5. Trait Anxiety Inventory 6. State Anxiety Inventory 7. Center for Epidemiologic Studies Depression Scale 8. Feetham Family Functioning Survey 9. Mental Adjustment Test	—	On health status	Stress from negative life events had small indirect effects on health status through self-esteem, parental competence, family functioning, mate relationship, and perceived support; model was supported with minor revisions
McNett (1987)	50 wheelchair-bound individuals recruited from 2 rehabilitation facilities	Cross-sectional, correlational, quantitative (LISREL analyses)	Lazarus & Folkman (1984) coping theory	—	1. Interpersonal Support Evaluation List 2. Questions concerning support effectiveness	1. Ways of Coping Checklist 2. McNett Coping Effectiveness Questionnaire	Negative direct effect on emotion-focused coping and a positive direct effect on problem-focused coping	—	Hypothesized causal model was supported by the results: perceived availability of SS, not use of SS, significantly and positively related to coping effectiveness through mediating variables of coping responses, emotion- and problem-focused

Swanson (1991)	20 women who had miscarried, 19 care providers in a newborn unit, and 8 young mothers receiving long-term public health intervention	Cross-sectional, qualitative, phenomenological, descriptive	Cobb (1976) view of SS with two nurse theories (Benner, 1984; Watson, 1979, 1985); middle-range theory of caring	—	—	Interview questions concerning caregiving	—	—	Five caring processes (knowing, being with, doing for, enabling, maintaining belief) were empirically described and a definition of caring was inductively derived; subdivisions of five processes identified to complete theory development and cross-validation with Watson & Benner
Yarcheski & Mahon (1989)	165 normal adolescents	Cross-sectional, quantitative, correlational (LISREL analyses to test causal model)	—	—	Personal Resource Questionnaire Part 2	1. Rosenberg Self-Esteem Scale 2. Personal Lifestyle Questionnaire	Direct effect on PHP and self-esteem	Indirect effect on PHP through self-esteem	Significant correlations between social support and positive health practices, self-esteem and PHP, age and PHP, and education and PHP; causal model needed modification because data from adolescents did not fit adult model

to test the construct itself, and to create new frameworks (Norbeck, 1991a). Support as a construct also has been interpreted by nurse theoreticians and applied to nursing theoretical frameworks.

❖ CHAPTER SIX ❖

Nursing Theory and Nurse Theoreticians

Significance of Social Support

Contributions of Nurses to Interpretation of the Social Support Construct

Conceptual models of social support, developed by nurse theoreticians, complementary to theory application and testing by nurse investigators (discussed in Chapter 5), have contributed to the interpretation of the construct of social support. Furthermore, the influence(s) of social support may be implicit in the theories of nursing. Hence a theory of nursing might be improved by explicitly incorporating considerations of social support, absent from extant theories.

Conceptual Models of Social Support Developed by Nurses

Although models have been developed by nurse theoreticians and researchers, almost all are based on and derived directly from theories advanced by psychologists. A review of 18 social support frameworks and models advanced in the nursing theoretical (not research) literature suggests that nursing's most laudable contribution to the conceptualization of social support has been to test, expand, elaborate, and explicate seminal theories and concepts. These theories occasionally are applied to specific target populations experiencing certain stressors. Thus Cronenwett and Kunst-Wilson (1981) employ House's (1981) paradigm of social support and stress in the context of a "transition to fatherhood paradigm"; Walker, MacBride, and Vachon (1977) apply Caplan's (1974) premises to their model of the support structure of the bereaved; and MacElveen-Hoehn and Eyres (1984) refer to Cobb (1976) in devising a model of social support for vulnerable children and families.

Sometimes several theorists' views are combined; Dimond and Jones (1983), for example, apply Weiss's (1974), Cobb's (1976), and Mitchell's (1969) fundamental social support and network concepts in developing their framework. This seems a reasonable approach, in view of the likelihood that no single theory of social support and social networks may be comprehensive. Clearly, however, no new theories of social support have been generated by nurse researchers. Attribution and equity theories have been virtually overlooked in nurse-developed theoretical frameworks, whereas coping theories predominate. Although Dimond (1985) concluded that "underlying most of the conceptualizations of social support is the assumption of reciprocity" (p. 7), this assumption is elusive in the definitions, typologies, and concepts included in the nonempirical nursing literature.

Norbeck and Tilden (1988) contribute to interpretation of the social support construct by summarizing shared assumptions concerning social support: (a) social support refers to interpersonal interactions and relationships, (b) these interactions provide emotional support or practical help, (c) the help usually is provided by members of the individual's social network, and (d) support is both given and received by network members. Their explication of assumptions augments the support-model development by nurses.

Relevance of Social Support to Extant Theoretical Frameworks for Nursing

Paradigmatic Origins of Nursing

Three main paradigms in the philosophy of science—the empirical-analytical, phenomenological or symbolic sciences, and critical social theory—have intersected nursing (Benner, 1985). The empirical, positivistic view claims that rational procedures for testing, validating, and rejecting hypotheses are required for scientific knowledge (Bernstern, 1976), and relies on mathematical logic for theory construction (Popkewitz, 1984). The phenomenological view reflects a "desire to bridge the gulf between ego consciousness and the social context" (Dallmayr & McCarthy, 1977). The goal of critical science is to demystify the patterns of knowledge and social conditions that restrict practical activities. The phenomenological acknowledgment of an interrelationship between the individual and society is congruent with social support and social network premises, whereas the critical sciences' focus on demystification merges with the self-help movement's aims (Chapter 2).

Regrettably, the empirical, positivistic tradition ignores political and social reality (Apple & Weiss, 1983), thereby reinforcing dominant societal values (Feinberg, 1983) and misrepresenting human action (Bernstein, 1976). For this reason there appears to be a shifting paradigm in professional practice, research, and education, away from dominance of scientific ideals to a personal, social, and holistic focus (Allender, 1986). Hence social-constructionist (Wright & Treacher, 1982) and holistic (Laura, 1985) views are beginning to receive attention as potential paradigms for health practitioners. Holistic conceptualizations of recipients are also emerging in nursing theories (Meleis, 1991).

Dissatisfactions with and decisions to reject one paradigm because of emerging anomalies, accompanied by the decision to accept a new paradigm, can lead to advances in professions (Charlesworth, 1982; Kuhn, 1970). The transfer of allegiance from paradigm to paradigm cannot be forced, and resistance to paradigm shifts will be encountered as long as some believe that the older paradigm will solve all the professional community's problems. It is difficult for health professionals to give up a dominant role reached through years of education, credentialism, and monopoly on practice areas. There is a threat to professional identity in addressing weaknesses and gaps in the professional sphere and in citizens becoming agents rather than targets of change. Individuals "who embrace a new paradigm at an early stage must often do so in defiance of the evidence . . . and have faith that the new paradigm will succeed with the many large problems that confront it knowing only that the older paradigm failed with a few" (Kuhn, 1970, p. 178).

However, nurses may be at the pre-paradigm stage, characterized by conflicting schools of thought; lack of agreement on theories, methodologies, and beliefs; and an evolutionary concern with development of conceptual frameworks. Therefore efforts at paradigmatic "change" or "creation" may encounter fewer obstacles than in other, more established disciplines. Further, there is an emerging belief in many disciplines that professionals are not confronted with exclusive choices in the selection of paradigms (Bernstein, 1976) and should not accept inappropriate restrictions in the range of paradigms that may legitimately be used (Susskind & Klein, 1985). The notion of professional paradigms acquired through education is pursued in Chapter 7.

The nursing discipline draws on theories and knowledge from the disciplines of psychology, sociology, and physiology. Three prototype theories in particular have been invoked as paradigmatic origins of nursing theory: symbolic interaction theory, developmental theory, and general systems theory. At this point the premises, concepts, and/or propositions of selected traditional models within each category are analyzed for potential relevance to social support.

Interaction Models

Several interaction models identify concepts and propositions potentially relevant to social support. The major concepts that the Riehl Interaction Model (Riehl, 1980) identifies are people, associations, social acts, interlinkages, role reversal, and the sick role. The only indirect reference that Riehl makes to social support is "intervention would require enlisting the aid of the family, friends and community resources to assist the patient through rehabilitation and back to a normal life" (Riehl, 1980, p. 355). Although she describes interactions as "reciprocal" and "complementary," Riehl exclusively emphasizes the individual patient and nurse roles and does not consider patients "to be really part of the health care system."

The Levine Interaction Model (Levine, 1971) identifies interaction, communication, and internal/external environment as concepts, and conservation of energy, structural integrity, personal integrity, and social integrity as principles. Illness is seen as a lonely, isolating event, which might be resolved by the participation of family. However, the principle of social integrity is given a minor place in the model and stops short of including other supportive individuals and lay groups in the community.

King (1981, 1986) employs the term *social* when describing human beings. Mutual goal setting is a promising component of her Open Systems Model and Goal Attainment Theory vis-à-vis social support. Although King stated that she did not follow the symbolic interaction school (Fawcett, 1989; Meleis, 1991), her conceptual model encompasses each of the characteristics of interaction models summarized by Fawcett (1989). Initially, King (1971, p. 23) conceived of "social systems" as groups of individuals joined together in a "network" or system of social relationships to achieve common goals. Unfortunately her 1981 definition restricts this system primarily to formal organizations, roles, and behaviors. Hence potential relevance to social support is diminished. When one considers the complexity of social systems and the necessity for nurses to assess and intervene at the aggregate and community levels, limitation of the conceptualization of "interpersonal systems" to individual-nurse interactions is regrettable.

Roy (1984) considers that human behavior represents adaptation to environmental and organismic forces. The environment encompasses external contextual and internal focal stimuli. However, Roy's Adaptation Model emphasizes environmental stressors rather than supports. Roy and Roberts (1981) refer to interdependence as "a comfortable balance in relationships with others." They identify the "interdependence mode" as the last of four modes of human adaptation to change (i.e., physiological needs, self-concept, role function, and interdependence). The interdependence mode includes reference to the "other" system, which is described as significant others (e.g., social affiliates, family members). Both Roy and King reflect a common inconsistency in nursing theories. Although they initially define nursing as care of individuals and groups, they subsequently confine discussion of nursing service to individuals.

Barnard's Child Health Assessment Interaction Theory is based on 10 theoretical assertions, several of which deal with caregiver-infant and parent-child interaction (Marriner-Tomey, 1989). Interaction is considered by Meleis (1991) to ideally incorporate both nurse/human being (client) interaction and human being/environment interaction. It is clear, however, that these interaction models emphasize the former to the virtual exclusion of the latter. Hence social support as a relevant concept has not been developed or even acknowledged by most interaction theorists.

Systems Models

Neuman's Systems Model has potential applicability in relation to social support. The environment, defined as consisting of internal and external forces that surround and influence humans and are influenced by humans, is not elaborated. Neuman's model emphasizes stressors in the environment. Johnson (1974, 1980) acknowledges social health and the social facets of individuals in her Behavioral Systems Model. However, she does not define either these concepts or the environment in that model.

More recent views of systems models also portray an embryonic evolution of interest in premises relevant to social support. For example, Bonnie Holaday (1987) modifies Johnson's model to emphasize the affiliative subsystem, whose goal is to relate or belong to something other than oneself, to achieve intimacy and inclusion, or to form cooperative and interdependent role relationships within human social systems. Duldt and Giffin (1985) defines systems communication as a dynamic process, involving continual adaptation and adjustment, between two or more human beings engaged in face-to-face interaction, but limits her discussion to the individual client-nurse interaction.

In sum, none of these systems theorists gives the social environment, affiliative subsystem, or interaction preeminence. They neither explicate these potentially relevant concepts nor expand their views to encompass the full array of socially supportive networks.

Developmental Models

Some facets of developmental models could be pertinent to nurses interested in developing theoretical frameworks based on social support. According to Rogers's Life Process Model, both human and environmental fields exist in a universe of open systems. As Clarke's (1986) review of this model clarifies, knowledge of life fields is vital for understanding relationships between living organisms. However, the focus of nursing roles is on "individual development" rather than the environment. Further, person-environment interaction tends to be limited to professional and institutional contexts.

One model, entitled Man-Living-Health, published in 1981 by Parse, draws on Rogers's model. Parse (1981) views humanity and the environment as constantly moving toward greater diversity through energy interchange. Environment is simplistically defined as all that humanity is not. Although the framework is considered broad enough in scope to be applicable to families in crisis or change by Marriner-Tomey (1989), other social networks are not included.

Orem (1980) identifies balance between solitude and social interaction as one of six universal self-care requisites. This theorist refers to the nurse providing a "supporting" environment. Proposition One states that "self-care and care of dependent family members are learned within the context of social groups by human interaction and communication" (Orem, 1980, p. 28). However, the focus is only on care of dependent family members and on nurses regulating the capability of patients to engage in self-care, rather than on potentiating supportive social networks and lay groups. Conceptualization of groups is restricted to the family, and that of environmental change is restricted to hospital and home environments. Nevertheless, active participation by clients in care is a positive feature of Orem's Self-Care Model.

Thus, developmental models focus on individuals, problems, and nursing functions. They retain an illness orientation and typically portray nurses as the final decision makers. Further, there is a limited view of environments and interaction.

Concepts

Considerable agreement exists that the central concepts constituting nursing conceptual models are the person (receiving nursing care), the environment (within which the person exists), the health-illness continuum (within which the person falls at the time of interaction with the nurse), and finally nursing (actions) (Conway, 1986; Cronenwett, 1983; Donaldson & Crowley, 1978; Ellis, 1982; Fawcett, 1989; Thibodeau, 1983). It is within the context of these four major components that theory development in nursing has proceeded. Theoretical differences in models relate to the emphasis placed on one or more of these components and to the way in which their relationships are viewed (Duldt & Giffin, 1985; Newman, 1983; Thibodeau, 1983).

Nursing

Theorists tend to define nursing by its goals, activities (Styles, 1982), attributes, process, tasks, and roles (Stanton, 1980; Stevens, 1984; Thibodeau, 1983). Divergent views of the numerous roles that nurses play were summarized by Torres (1986) and Meleis (1991). Not one of the theorists they cited referred to the possibility of an indirect consultant or partnership role for the nurse (considered appropriate to working with informal support networks). The "expert" role, in its varying forms, received the most attention.

Defining nursing with "nursing" can be confusing and circular. In nursing theory, the nature of nursing is generally represented as helping. The primary focus is on the interpersonal interactions occurring between nurse and client (Chinn & Jacobs, 1987). However, conceptualizations of nursing that focus on the interpersonal process have not adequately formulated specific goals that enlighten us about nursing as a distinctive form of helping (Ellis, 1982). Some might consider the concept of "caring" as a reasonable substitute for "nursing," but this appears to be a more limited interpretation than "helping," a prevalent concept in social support theory.

Person/Individual/Client

Most nursing models conceptualize individuals holistically, as more than the sum of that person's biological, sociological, and psychological parts (Chinn & Jacobs, 1987; Stanton, 1980). The concept of "person," in the nursing conceptual models and metaparadigm, delineates the recipient, client, or beneficiary of nursing services, from varying conceptual perspectives. For example, people may be seen as active or reactive beings who cooperate with, compete with, influence, or are influenced by the environment (Thibodeau, 1983).

In the social sciences literature, Bernstein (1976, p. 96) refers to the concept of a "person" as being important. Regrettably the conceptualization of client and person is generally limited to the individual level. As Chopoorian (1986) claims, nursing's paradigm has led to the production of roles largely confined to individualized, privatized spheres of care.

Health

Wellness and illness may be conceptualized as a continuum, as coexistent states, or as mutually exclusive states (Thibodeau, 1983). The concept of health is most often viewed as a health-illness continuum. However, some nursing scholars reject the health-illness continuum and view health as a phenomenon that is not linked only to the presence or absence of illness (Chinn, 1983; Stevens, 1984).

Currently, nursing models emphasize the concept of health (Newman, 1983; Smith, 1981). Some theorists view the health process as interdependent with circumstances in the environment. Others, on the other hand, inadequately view the health process as something that originates with or can be achieved largely by the individual.

Environment

Most nursing models focus on a selected aspect of the environment (Ellis, 1982; Thibodeau, 1983). The environment is seen as a source of stressors in most models, rather than a source of resources (Fawcett, 1989). Nursing care can encompass manipulation of the environment and of environment-person interactions (Ellis, 1982; Meleis, 1991). Furthermore, nursing actions are created, developed, modified, and constrained within a given environmental context (Kim, 1983b). Therefore the environment is an essential component for theoretical thinking in nursing.

However, with few exceptions, even though it is a central element in the nursing paradigm, nurse theorists have not clearly articulated nor elaborated upon the concept of environment (Chinn & Jacobs, 1987; Chopoorian, 1986; Flaskerud & Halloran, 1980; Meleis, 1991). "With the individual as the focus for nursing interventions, the environment, as a complex set of structures and relationships, fades into the periphery of nursing's attention and is not treated as an arena for action" (Chopoorian, 1986, p. 42). Frequently nursing deals with people who are experiencing, anticipating, or completing transitions that are situational, developmental, or health-illness events (Meleis, 1991). Nursing should not isolate the transition of an individual, a family, or a community from the environment. Clearly the concept of environment must become prominent in nursing theory. Chopoorian (1986) comments: "To understand the dilemmas and issues that influence human beings and hence create conditions for health or illness, nurses must reach beyond the privatized concerns of the individual to the surrounding world for explanation and action" (p. 53).

A few critics of this latter deficiency proposed tentative approaches to conceptualizing the environment. Kim (1983b) classified the environment as spatial, temporal, or qualitative (physical, symbolic, or social). Social environment, in this typology, refers to individuals and groups with whom a person interacts and communicates, and encompasses social support. Chopoorian (1986, p. 47) suggests reconceptualization of environment as social, economic, and political structures and as human social relations.

Stevens (1989) responds to Chopoorian's (1986) challenge to create a more comprehensive view of the environment and its interaction with persons and health. She employs critical social theory to expand the understanding of environment by critically analyzing the social, economic, and political worlds of nursing events. "The oppressive social structures that constrain a person's health, limit their life possibilities, and restrict their . . . participation in society" (Stevens, 1989, p. 63) are critiqued. Collective experiences and group interactions with the environment are acknowledged (Stevens, 1989), although neither social support nor a new model or definition of the environment are proffered.

Concepts from sociological models as well as nursing models may function well in the environment domain of a conceptual framework (Kim, 1983a; Reed, 1986). Theories centering on the environment could describe environmental properties, components, and dimensions that help maintain and promote health (Meleis, 1991). In sum, the environment is a greatly neglected concept in nursing conceptual models. However, some preparatory groundwork has been laid in recent years. The time is ripe for explication, elaboration, and application of this critical concept, primarily in its social domain.

Summary of Linkage of Nursing Theory and Social Support Theory

The environment theme (which is particularly relevant to social support and social networks) is given limited attention in traditional conceptual models of nursing. No nursing theorists concentrated on groups or the community, and only a few consider the family. Furthermore, Nightingale (classified as an early environment theorist) focused only on the physical environment rather than the social environment. Other nurse theorists typically emphasize stressors in the environment rather than supports. However, Barnard describes the environment as "supporting" (Marriner-Tomey, 1989). Finally, the perspective of the consumer does not consistently enter into nursing models. Although most conceptual models in nursing refer to person-environment interaction, consideration usually is limited to nurse-patient interactions. Conceptual models do not typically address the potential relevance of social support or lay aggregate and community helping in anything other than a superficial sense.

Recent applications of these traditional nursing models and development of new models, however, illustrate attempts to integrate social support. Swanson's (1991) development of a middle-range theory of caring is compared not only to Watson's (1979, 1985) nursing "carative" factors and Benner's (1984) delineation of the helping role of the nurse, but also to Cobb's (1976) definition of social support. The "Theory of Caring" (see Table 5.4) encompasses five processes—knowing, being with, doing for, enabling, and maintaining belief—in which the carer/provider and recipient are engaged. Only "enabling," however, includes informing, supporting, and validating—illustrative of the functions of social support. Swanson (1991) claims that "although caring is most likely an aspect of all supportive relationships, not all caring relationships are experienced as social support" because mutual obligation is lacking.

Tulman and Fawcett (1990) conceptualize functional status during pregnancy in terms of Roy's Adaptation Model (1984) and role theory. They include a discussion of the positive relationship found by nurse investigators between social support and adjustment during childbearing (Brown, 1986a; Norbeck & Tilden, 1983; Tulman & Fawcett, 1990). Marital relationships were associated with transition to parenthood (Tulman & Fawcett, 1990) that links concepts from Roy's model with health, individual psychosocial, and family variables—the last encompass social support from family and friends and quality of the marital relationship.

Travelbee's Theory of Nursing (1971) was used as a framework for a support group of nurses created to discuss changing job roles, offer support, and learn problem-solving skills (Cook, 1990). The theory, originally developed for interaction with individuals, was adapted to group work—perhaps because of the emphasis on finding meaning, empathy, and rapport.

Fruehwirth (1989) applied Johnson's model in assessment and intervention with a support group for caregivers of persons with Alzheimer's disease. Johnson's model was used as a guide to identify and interpret behavior changes. Although not clarified by Fruehwirth, the affiliative and sexual subsystems could be related to social support. Social isolation, decreased coping, lack of intimacy, and desire for support from family were identified as "goal" or "set," and attending the support group as an appropriate "action."

Nevertheless, despite their exploratory applications, Tulman and Fawcett (1990), Cook (1990), and Fruehwirth (1989) do not explicitly link social support theory to a nursing theory. In contrast, Frey (1989) empirically tested a theoretical formulation of social support, family health, and child health derived from King's conceptual framework. Social support was conceptualized from King's concept of interaction within the interpersonal system. Frey maintains that definitions of social support (Cobb, 1976; House, 1981; Kahn & Antonucci, 1980) are consistent with interaction as described by King. The finding that parents' social support was linked to family health was interpreted as evidence of the interacting relationship between interpersonal (social support) and social (family) systems ("King's terminology"). The author contended that the study supported King's conceptual framework and extended the interpretation of social support. This is the sole explicit linkage of social support theory and nursing theory.

Anticipated Amenability of the Nursing Profession to a Social Support Theoretical Framework

There is beginning recognition by nursing-theory analysts of the potential merits of social support research and theories. Fawcett (1989) cites Barnard, Snyder, and Spletz's (1984) investigation of social support as evidence of evolving exemplars in nursing. Meleis (1991) identifies Norbeck (1981) as an example of an author who viewed nursing via another paradigm. Norbeck (1982) attempts a linkage between social support and nursing practice. She delineated six theoretical assumptions in her model for clinical research. Norbeck (1981), like Dimond and Jones (1983), argued that properties of the person and of the situation jointly determine need for social support and actual support available. Finally, Fawcett (1989) invoked the social support literature to exemplify descriptive, explanatory, and predictive theories.

Environmental social support is a significant concept for nursing practice because nurses, in conjunction with clients, can assess the factors that contribute to enacted and perceived support (see Chapter 4). Social support mediates the relationship between life stress and health status. Although a comprehensive theory of social support has not yet evolved, operationalization of the construct and hypotheses regarding its impact on health have developed, and nurses have contributed to this process. For example, Norbeck et al. (1981), drawing on Kahn and Antonucci (1980), operationalized three forms of social support: aid, affirmation, and affect. Norbeck (1985b) later devised a simplified model of the indirect, direct, and interactive relationships between stress, social support, and health outcomes. Although international research is needed to test whether social support is a universal construct for all cultures, social support theory development should guide nursing practice (Norbeck & Tilden, 1988).

Nurse educators may be beginning to respond to the challenge of integrating social support theory into educational curricula. Tilden (1985b) provided a descriptive analysis of the frequency and type of theories about social support that were incorporated into the curricula of the undergraduate and graduate programs of one university school of nursing in the United States. Tilden (1985b) cautions that "the report should not be considered representative nor conclusive, but only suggestive of trends" (p. 7). Hilbert and Allen (1985) demonstrated a positive impact of social support on the self-esteem of nursing students (see also Chapter 7).

Thus the stage is set in the research (a detailed review is included in Chapter 5), theoretical, practice, and educational spheres of the nursing profession for a conceptual model derived from social support theories. However, prevalent assumptions, concepts, and relationship statements need to be reinterpreted because consumer and lay network viewpoints are rarely represented in nursing theories. A theory of nursing should be developed that merges selected facets of the interactionism and systems models. Logically, this could be based on social support theories and relevant supplementary theories.

Social Support
Conceptual Framework for Nursing

Unlike its predecessors, the proposed conceptual framework encompasses a social focus, emphasizes the consumer, explicates the environment domain, and acknowledges client-environment interaction (Stewart, 1990c).

Assumptions

Sixteen assumptions underlie the proposed framework. They reflect premises concerning the nature of human beings, their environments, health and health care, and nursing that are consistent with the perspective of a social or primary health care model rather than that of a medical model. These assumptions are (Stewart, 1990c):

1. Persons are social, rational, perceiving, thinking beings.
2. Persons have unique knowledge bases derived from personal life experiences.
3. Persons are holistic, biopsychosocial, cultural, spiritual beings.
4. Persons have the right and the responsibility to seek optimum health for themselves.
5. Persons are competent to help themselves and others.
6. Persons have the right to independent choice and control with respect to help from their environments and from professional nurses.
7. Persons' perceptions of support from their social environments may differ from perceptions of nurses and network members.
8. The environment serves as a source of diverse forms of support as well as stress.
9. Environmental support has a positive impact on health and health behavior of persons.
10. Health has social, psychological, and physiological facets.
11. Nursing is concerned with persons, their environments, and their health.
12. Nursing focuses on promotion, maintenance, and restoration of health and prevention of illness.
13. Primary health care by nurses and social support from environments both encompass lay helping.
14. Nursing deals with individuals, families, groups, communities, and social systems.
15. Nursing services are offered in a variety of community-based settings.
16. Nursing's knowledge base encompasses integrated conceptual, critical, interpersonal, and technical competencies derived from formal education and informal experiences.

Concepts

Changed Interpretation of Nursing Metaparadigm Concepts

The four concepts of the nursing metaparadigm were necessarily defined to reflect an altered philosophy of professional partnership with lay helping networks. Definitions of environment, health, nursing, and person developed for this conceptual framework are presented below.

Environment. The context of nursing's beneficiaries and services. It is social-psychological (consisting of natural and created social networks, which are sources of support as well as stress), political-economic (including social movements such as the mutual-aid self-help and consumerism movements), and physical (encompassing not only institutional settings but also diverse community-based sites).

Health. A proportional composite of the social, psychological, physical, and spiritual well-being of individuals, families, groups, and communities, which must be promoted, maintained, and restored. Social health is determined by embeddedness in a social network or integration within the community.

Nursing. A helping profession, with the goals of promoting, maintaining, and restoring the health of individuals, families, groups, and communities and of facilitating self-help and client-environment interaction (mutual aid). Nursing equally encompasses primary health care, consultant, liaison, educator, advocate (empowerment), and care-provider roles. Nurses can collaborate as partners with beneficiaries and their actual or potential informal helping networks and with members of other health disciplines. Nurses indirectly mobilize and enhance support during periods of stress, crisis, or transition. The utilization of nursing services is influenced by the social networks of beneficiaries.

Focal Persons. Individuals, families, groups, or communities that have unitary social, psychological, spiritual, and physical characteristics.

They participate as partners with nurses in promoting, maintaining, and restoring their health. Focal persons continuously and mutually interact with their environments, while seeking independence and interdependence.

Core Concepts Related to Metaparadigm Concepts

Core concepts were selected to be compatible with the nursing metaparadigm and to reflect concepts congruent with social support drawn from the social-psychological literature. Accordingly, 20 concepts (highlighted in italics) were derived from pertinent theories to elucidate the environment, health, focal person, and nursing domains (Stewart, 1990c).

Environment. Social support concepts can be operationally classified as social embeddedness, perceived social support, and enacted support (Chapter 1). Enacted and perceived *social support* can be described and interpreted from the distinct, yet often interlocking, theoretic viewpoints of *attribution, social comparison, social exchange, social interaction,* social learning (*collective efficacy, experiential knowledge*), and social movements (*empowerment*).

Health. Confirmation of the direct (main) and indirect (buffering) effects of environmental social support on physical and mental health is central to this conceptual framework for nursing. Intuitively, social support's positive impact on social and spiritual health of focal persons also could be surmised. Several empirical studies investigate preventive functions of social support. Social support influences susceptibility to some infections and some aspects of the immune response. The one concept that appears to be especially pertinent to the health promotion and primary preventive traits of social support is *immunocompetence.*

Nursing. Collaboration and *consultant, helping, partner,* and *primary health care* roles are assumed to be congruent with social support premises and with nursing. Furthermore, *professional nursing knowledge* needs to be conceptualized in a framework for nursing.

Focal Person. Coping, loneliness, self-esteem, and *self-care/self-help* concepts are pertinent to social support from the focal-person perspective.

Relationship Statements

The proposed relationship statements are correlational (not causal), linking subconcepts and concepts between or within the four metaparadigm components. The relationships are based primarily on linkages uniquely developed for this framework (Stewart, 1990c). Although most concepts were redefined rather than created, the relationship statements are newly developed, because (with the exception of the buffering and main hypotheses) the parent theory (social support) lacked specific propositions relevant to health care.

This social support framework leaves the relationships among the four nursing metaparadigm components—"Nursing studies the wholeness or health of humans, recognizing that humans are in continuous interaction with their environment" (Fawcett, 1989, p. 5)—basically unchanged, but emphasizes the interaction of focal persons with their social-cultural environment and the appropriate role of the nurse. The first relationship statement links all four components in this framework. The remaining statements relate theories pertinent to social support to specific metaparadigm concepts.

1. Nurses consulting with focal persons and members of their support network can enhance physical, psychological, and social health and promote positive health behaviors of focal persons.
2. Nurse consultation with focal persons facilitates focal persons' interaction with their social network and facilitates self-care.
3. If there is external attribution of the cause of the focal person's health problems or concerns and internal attribution of the relevant problem solutions by the support network and the nurse, then help sought from and rendered by the social network or the nurse will be effective.
4. If the attribution of causes and solutions of the health concerns by focal persons, support network members, and nurses are congruent, then help available from and enacted by the support network or the nurse will be effective.
5. If the natural network of the focal persons has been depleted through bereavement, divorce, or other loss, loneliness may occur and may increase susceptibility to health problems through decreased immunocompetence. Conversely, health problems may instigate network losses.
6. The nurse may mitigate or prevent health problems associated with loneliness from depleted or deficient social-network support by

mobilizing created networks, by enhancing natural networks, or by temporarily supplementing with nursing support.

7. Social support from natural or created networks can help focal persons cope with stress and prevent health problems.
8. The nurse can, through consultation, encourage upward social comparison in dyadic or group-level support networks, which may enhance coping and health maintenance by the focal person.
9. The nurse can, through consultation, promote reciprocal exchange of support between focal persons and their natural or created social network, which may in turn enhance the focal person's self-esteem and the effectiveness of helping.
10. The nurse's interaction with both the focal person and the social network increases collaboration and in turn enhances helping and coping effectiveness.
11. Reciprocal exchange of information derived from the nurse's professional knowledge, the social network's lay or experiential knowledge, and the focal person's experiential knowledge should promote partnership role assumption by each party.
12. Experiential knowledge and expertise of lay help movements may be in conflict with professional knowledge and competence acquired by nurses and hence must be respected and accorded equal status if nurse-social network collaboration and partnership are to occur.
13. Collaborative partnership roles can be learned when there is negotiation among equal parties regarding respective goals, responsibilities, role expectations, and status in interactions among nurses, focal persons, and social networks.
14. Joint assumption of partner roles by nurses with focal persons and with members of the natural or created support network facilitates assumption of primary health care roles by nurses.
15. Nurses' assumption of primary health care roles promotes the health of focal persons.
16. The nurse can, through consultation, facilitate resocialization of focal persons and their support networks from traditional, passive patient role expectations (by society and professionals) to new, partner roles.
17. Feedback regarding the nurse's professional helping from focal persons and from social-network members should enhance the effectiveness of that helping.
18. Feedback from focal persons regarding lay helping by social-network members should increase the effectiveness of such lay helping.

19. Interaction between the three open systems—nurse, focal person, and lay support network—as partners constitutes a form of systemic linkage.
20. The interaction between focal persons and their created social environment promotes social learning (and hence empowerment and collective efficacy). This learning can be facilitated by nurses acting in consultant roles to enhance positive health behaviors.

These 20 relationship statements, together with the corresponding relationship figure, constitute the evolutionary theory base.

Model

The complete conceptual model based on social support (Stewart, 1990c) is schematically depicted in Figure 6.1, in the form of connecting blocks. Within each block, representing the four nursing metaparadigmatic concepts, all subconcepts or core concepts are classified. In keeping with the philosophical thrust of the model, the terms "helper role" and "partner role" recur in the focal-person, environment, and nursing domains. In addition, unique forms of knowledge and respective attributions are pertinent to each domain. The interactions (interaction models), feedback, and systemic linkages (systems models) between nursing metaparadigmatic domains are represented by arrows. Although the helping role is conceptually grounded in caring (Swanson, 1991) and collaborative decision making has been conceptualized by Kim (1983a), neither role is defined operationally in either the nursing or social support literature. Operational definitions for helping and partner roles, therefore, follow:

- A facilitative helping role is accompanied by the belief that focal persons are strong and are deprived yet deserving of help, and that assistance should be temporary, should result in enhanced opportunity and self-actualization for the focal person, and can come from the focal person, peer members in the social network, or professionals. (This belief combines facets of the compensatory, moral, and enlightenment models [Brickman et al., 1982]. In contrast, the traditional medical model is accompanied by the view that focal persons are ill and weak, that donors are expert professionals, and that help is indefinite and should result in cure.)

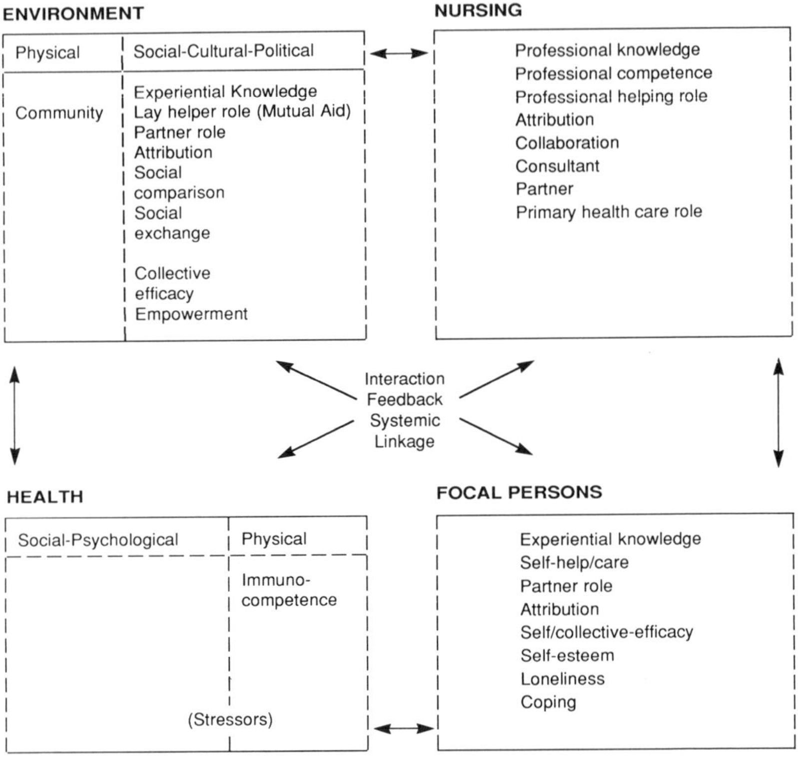

Figure 6.1. Nursing Education Conceptual Model Based on Social Support

- A partner role is demonstrated by the frequency with which there is joint exchange of information and joint decision making regarding goals and methods to achieve goals among nurses, focal persons, and their families, friends, or self-help groups; mutual working to achieve these goals; and joint evaluation of effectiveness of emotional and physical health outcomes. A partner role is further demonstrated by the degree to which observable and perceived equality exists in levels of status, control, and responsibility in these relationships.

Summary

Nurses have generated conceptual models to administer and elucidate the construct of social support; however, no new theories have been created and pertinent social-psychological theories have not been invoked. Nursing reflects a shift to a phenomenological, holistic paradigm, more consistent with acknowledgment of clients' networks. In fact, its models represent three paradigmatic origins—symbolic interaction, developmental, and systems theory. Yet the environment that encompasses social networks, the interactions between clients and their networks, and the interactions of nurses with these networks have not been explicated conceptually. Accordingly, a social or primary health care model for nursing is proposed. This model was later tested at McMaster University School of Nursing (Sword, Noesgaard, & Majumdar, 1992).

There is an emerging view that there is merit in theoretic pluralism for nursing (Meleis, 1991), rather than a single theory or model as earlier nursing theorists urged. Most disciplines have a single metaparadigm but multiple conceptual models (Fawcett, 1989). Thus the new conceptual framework, rather than being a complete replacement, would be applied in addition to existing models developed by nurses. Concepts from several non-nursing theories were integrated and adapted in this alternative nursing framework.

The theoretic framework proffers a new way of approaching nursing care and illuminates lay helping phenomena. The proposed framework is consistent with international intentions to institute widespread primary health care. As A. F. Meleis comments, "I wonder how different would nursing theories be if we adopt primary health care as the major (or only) strategy for delivery of nursing care" (personal communication, 1987).

❖ CHAPTER SEVEN ❖

Nursing Education
Significance of Social Support

Issues relevant to the education of all professionals, such as professional socialization, and matters specific to the education of nurses are deliberated in this chapter.

Professional Knowledge Regarding Lay Helpers

Interviews and surveys of professionals working with mutual-aid self-help groups and of self-help group members (reported in Chapter 2) reveal a prevalent perception of a professional knowledge gap. Professional knowledge was found to be strongly associated with referrals to and linkages with self-help groups (Miller, 1983) and with supportive attitudes toward group development (Black & Drachman, 1985). However, the vast majority of professionals reported little or no coverage in their educational programs, rated their current knowledge as either fair or poor, and desired further information about such groups (Black & Drachman, 1985; Farquharson, 1987; Farquharson & Cardinal, 1989; Levy, 1978; Todres, 1982; Toseland & Hacker, 1985). Both professionals and members also identified role ambiguity as a problem. Subsequent revelation of complementary roles by comparative studies of professional and natural helpers (e.g., Toro, 1986; Toseland, 1990; Toseland, Rossiter, Peak, & Hill, 1990; Tracey & Toro, 1989) could elucidate this uncertainty.

These studies, however, did not solicit nurses' views. The World Health Organization (1985) exhorts "nursing . . . schools to include in their educational programs the philosophy of health for all, the principles of primary health care" (p. 158). Given that mutual aid is an important vehicle of primary health care and health promotion and given that nurses are a particularly appropriate group of health professionals to implement these service forms, it is timely to examine nurses' preparedness to advance health promotion and primary health care through linkage with lay help groups.

Nurses' Views and Experiences

To elicit information about nurses' attitudes, knowledge, and experiences regarding self-help groups, questionnaires were mailed to 200 randomly selected hospital nurses and to all 177 community health nurses working in metropolitan Halifax, Nova Scotia (Stewart, 1989a). The majority were able to identify characteristics and benefits that reflected common definitions of self-help groups. Nevertheless, almost all respondents viewed their relevant level of knowledge as only fair and the most commonly cited reason for nonreferral to groups was lack of information, comparable to findings for other professions (Black & Drackman, 1985; Miller, 1985; Toseland & Hacker, 1985). Yet Farquharson and Cardinal (1989) accentuate effective referrals in professional practice with lay supporters. Nurses' wishes to learn community organization, group work, and consultation skills reflect perceptions of other disciplines (Black & Drackman, 1985; Farquharson, 1987; Farquharson & Cardinal, 1989; Jacobs & Goodman, 1989; Miller, 1985).

Twice as many nurses attended group meetings to increase their familiarity with self-help groups as served initiator, speaker, consultant, or nonprofessional member roles. Yet fewer held any of these roles than other professionals (see Chapter 2). The three roles nurses preferred most for professionals were referral agent, consultant, and liason, comparable to other disciplines. Nurses favored the initiator/creator role less (both in attitude and in practice) than did members of other disciplines studied elsewhere. This directive role is a subject of controversy. There is an emerging view that it should be temporary if instituted at all. Almost 70% made frequent or occasional referrals, exceeding rates reported for other disciplines.

Almost all nurses held positive attitudes regarding the effectiveness, merits, and functions of self-help groups; professional linkage with self-help groups; and their future personal involvement. In fact, few perceived conflict or tension between professionals and members and almost all valued lay help, even if professionals were not present. In contrast, Toseland and Hacker (1982, 1985) discovered a unanimous preference among social workers for referring only to those groups that encompassed professional involvement.

The nurses welcomed pertinent education and information in a variety of forms, and acknowledged that lack of knowledge/information is a major barrier for those who do not refer. The fact that respondents seldom assumed roles for which they were attitudinally ready may reflect the passive position of some nurses with respect to other disciplines, the lack of formal agency relationships with self-help groups, or the perceived need for germane skill development and information. It is difficult to determine whether this is due to real or perceived lack of opportunity (Stewart, 1989a).

Over half of the nurses surveyed viewed experiential knowledge and role models (social learning concepts) as characteristics of mutual-aid groups. The ability to give as well as to receive aid (indicative of exchange theory premises) is valued highly by lay-group members (Gottlieb, 1982a; Levy, 1978; Marques, 1983) and recognized by almost all nurses (96%). Nurses' beliefs that self-help group aid complements professional services and provides a unique service illustrate balance theory concepts. Although lack of information does not necessarily imply need for information, evolving citizen demand in the form of social movements dictates that nurses as health professionals be knowledgeable and prepared. In this context, it is significant that nurses rarely recognized the peer-control and social-action elements of mutual-aid groups. (These theories were discussed in Chapters 1 and 2.)

The foregoing suggests the need for nursing education in appropriate knowledge, roles, skills, and attitudes. Indeed, the World Health Organization (WHO) (1984, 1985) recommended changes in professional training, internationally and nationally, to enable health professionals to develop knowledge and understanding of self-help groups. Hence pertinent content should be included in health-professional curricula. If one function of a curriculum is to teach students about professional practice and thereby to improve the quality of professional praxis, there is a need to assess curriculum content to determine whether appropriate didactic and experiential elements are incorporated.

A few successful examples of curricula that achieve this WHO goal, to a greater or lesser extent, are emerging. However, none of these curricula or programs has been empirically evaluated according to short- or long-term modification of roles, knowledge, attitudes, and skills. Nevertheless, the self-help literature reflects a predominant emphasis on social-worker education and on physician preparation (Bremer-Schulte, 1983; Farquharson & Cardinal, 1989; Goetzel, Shelow, & Croen, 1983; Gottlieb & Farquharson, 1985; Traunstein, 1984). The single largest health-professional group that might interact with and contribute to self-help groups—nurses—has been overlooked.

Nurse Educators' Views

Initial basic education of nurses at the undergraduate level about the role and impact of lay helping and support networks and about appropriate professional roles and relationships with these networks thus appears advisable; however, only one nursing program that encompassed some social-support relevant content has been briefly outlined by Tilden (1985b). Accordingly, the purpose of this descriptive study was to identify curricular content in Canadian university schools of nursing germane to lay support groups (Stewart, 1988).

Most curricula included some of the theories pertinent to lay support groups but overlooked the relevance of others. The virtual absence of social comparison theories seems incongruent with the fact that in most curricula self-help groups were identified as points of reference or comparison with peers. The premises of reciprocity or equity theories, so relevant to mutual-aid groups, were addressed only by a minority of the schools, according to these respondents. The most commonly identified benefit was experience sharing, although experiential knowledge and social learning theories were less often included in curricula. Only half described the self-help group as a coping aid, despite the fact that all curricula include stress and coping theories. Finally, the minimal recognition of these groups' appraisal support function reflects the infrequent inclusion of attribution theories that interpret appraisal. Thus instruction regarding practice sometimes may be inadequately grounded in theory. On the other hand, there may not be uniformity in understanding the conceptualization and characteristics of lay support groups.

The most frequently cited benefits of self-help groups that were relayed in curricula were emotional support, opportunity to share experiences, and informational support. Although other disciplines recognize the primary benefit of emotional support, they also emphasize normalization and decreased stigmatization (Miller, 1983; Toseland & Hacker, 1985; Tracey & Toro, 1989). In contrast, self-help group members, though acknowledging the benefits of shared experience and informational support, perceive reciprocal or bidirectional help as the greatest benefit of membership (Kurtz, 1984; Romeder, 1982).

There could be increased experiential emphasis on the natural tensions between professionals and nonprofessionals and on professional partnership relationships with lay helpers and support groups. Regrettably, less than one third of the curricula included the partnership relationship and determination of appropriate professional roles as clinical assignments. In contrast, many of the roles frequently identified in the classroom could be categorized as indirect partner roles rather than direct or directive provider roles. However, nursing curricula rarely communicated the referral role, which is unfortunate given the frequent identification of this role in self-help group studies (see Chapter 2) and its reported omission in nursing practice (e.g., Field & Renfrew, 1991). The most commonly conveyed professional role, the consultant role, is also emphasized by other disciplines and self-help group members (Cherniss & Cherniss, 1987; Gottlieb, 1982a; Toseland & Hacker, 1985).

The traditional focus of nursing education on developing group work and leadership skills, rather than on community organization and consultant skills, is perhaps misplaced in light of the skills reinforced in the social support literature. For example, Black and Drachman (1985) found that social workers required educational preparation in group work and community organization skills for work with support groups. Group stability, growth, and innovation were associated with consultation between mutual-aid group members and professionals (Cherniss & Cherniss, 1987).

The predominant mixture of didactic and experiential learning experiences in nursing curricula reflects educational recommendations in the self-help group literature (Bremer-Schulte, 1983; Gottlieb

& Farquharson, 1985). However, observation and assessment were more frequently used as learning experiences than role playing, videotaping, and direct role implementation (Stewart, 1988). "Passive" observation of self-help group meetings also was the most prevalent form of professional nurses' contact with self-help groups (Stewart, 1989a). One sixth of the schools employed videotaped role-playing sessions as a teaching technique, which have also been incorporated in the one documented curriculum for social workers (Gottlieb & Farquharson, 1985). Nevertheless, given the paucity of information on social work and medical curricula about self-help groups, and given the fact that what has been reported has not been evaluated, these comparisons may not be useful.

Finally, the fact that 71% of the 26 responding schools reportedly include some content relevant to mutual-aid and support groups in their undergraduate curricula is encouraging in light of the World Health Organization (1985) recommendation referred to earlier. Yet relevant continuing education courses offered by a logical vehicle, university schools of nursing, are virtually nonexistent in the country, in spite of the probable need (Stewart, 1988).

* * *

In short, despite the sampling problems and selective focus on support groups only (rather than all manifestations of support), these two studies of nurse practitioners and educators reveal attitudinal readiness and educational deficiencies in requisite role preparation as consultants and partners.

Attitude and Role Modification Through Education: Transition From Provider to Partner

Students who enter professional training programs in the health fields typically come from a middle-class culture, which socializes them to believe that "expert solutions take precedence over experiential solutions" (Gottlieb & Farquharson, 1985). Such early ingrained attitudes (which have cognitive and affective dimensions) frequently resist challenge and change. Further, attitudes that relate to the professional ideology and that have become internalized as part of the ego identity of the practitioner are relatively slow to alter (Jarvis, 1983). The person entering a profession embarks on an enculturation process that includes more than the mastery of theoretical knowledge, because it emphasizes attitudes and role behavior. Moving to a conception of consumers as partners runs counter to the health professional's traditional understanding of the helping process and of professional roles. This fundamental shift in attitudes is complex and will necessitate much more than theoretical, didactic curricular change. Educational approaches to attitudinal change must elicit the attention and comprehension of the individual. Faculty commitment to the revised ideology of professional practice and experiential opportunities to practice pertinent skills and roles are also required.

The evolution of consumer and self-help movements (discussed in Chapter 2) challenges professionals to transform traditional roles and ideologies from expert provider of services to partner. As self-help groups acquire autonomy and as the professional role changes from expert provider to invited catalyst or consultant, learning must occur. However, the traditional model of professional training frequently is geared at the direct-service role, creating problems of role strain during the transition to the "indirect" collegial, consultant role. In fact, professional education programs are based on an ideology of professionalism and socialization into professional values.

Professionalism and Professional Socialization

The sociological theories of professionalism could enable analysis of the relationship between professional and lay systems. Yet, Dingwall and Lewis (1983) and Friedson (1983) purport that little theoretical work has been done in the sociology of professions on the "fit" of lay helpers and self-help with the formal system. Professional socialization is considered to be an interactive process whereby the professional culture and ideology are transmitted initially through an educational process, leading to the acquisition of requisite knowledge, skills, values, and roles (Jarvis, 1983; McCain, 1985; McKinlay 1982; Stark, Lowther, Hagerty, & Orczyk, 1986) and to "internalization of standards defined by the profession's elite" (Larson, 1977).

Bledstein (1976) maintains that professionalism is a set of learned values that reinforce the public's consciousness of dependence and vulnerability. The monopoly of professionals over "necessary" skills and knowledge derives from special training (Jarvis, 1983; Lenrow &

Cowden, 1980; Miller, 1983). The social significance of professional knowledge in reproducing a particular order (Dingwall & Lewis, 1983) and maintaining a protective mystique (Reuschemeyer, 1983) has been reaffirmed. Schon (1987) ironically depicts the traditional view of professional knowledge as "I am presumed to know and must claim to do so, regardless of my own uncertainty." A consequence of this professionalization of knowledge, however, is to make laypersons more dependent upon experts in society (Popkewitz, 1984).

Rather than manipulation, hostility, or indifference, professionals need to learn a partnership orientation to consumers and laypersons that, in Larson's (1977) words, "challenges the division between professionals and laity." New competencies (which imply changed knowledge, skills, and attitudes) should be developed in educational programs. Two competencies described by Stark et al. (1986) as outcomes of health professional education could be considered particularly relevant to professional preparation for working with consumers and lay helpers. *Contextual* competence is an understanding of the broad social, economic, and cultural setting in which the profession is practiced, and *adaptive* competence is the ability to adjust to new conditions in a rapidly changing society. Farquharson and Cardinal's (1989) "Competency profile for human service professionals working with self help mutual-aid groups" explicates germane domains of competence: (a) establish effective communications; (b) understand and value self-help and mutual-aid; (c) learn from and apply experiential know-how; and (d) support the strength of mutual aid. Clearly these new competencies differ from those reinforced by traditional professional socialization.

Professional Paradigms

Kuhn (1970) raises the question of professional socialization in the context of "paradigms" (discussed in Chapter 6), which are composed of disciplinary matrices. Disciplinary matrices are acquired implicitly through modeling and shared exemplars in the educational process (Eckberg & Hill, 1979; Kuhn, 1977). Students are taught to learn and accept the paradigm (Jacox, 1981) revealed in its textbooks, lectures, and laboratory sessions.

An educational process is one approach to early socialization of professionals away from the traditional mode. Rather than making them more "expert," as early versions of the sociology of professions would suggest, this reprofessionalization could facilitate attitudinal, knowledge, and skill changes that are more amenable to partnership with lay participants. However, educators must remember that socialization activities directed toward the development of a professional identity are not always consciously undertaken. For example, faculty may reflect different, if not conflicting, paradigms, particularly if the conceptual framework for curricular reform has not been accepted. As Cherniss and Cherniss (1987) contend, "professionals should recognize that their training and socialization may lead them to overly restrict the universe of service alternatives" (or paradigms).

Summary

In summary, there are numerous potentiating and limiting forces (see Figure 7.1) within nursing and society that would influence the impact of educational strategies for professional change: specifically, consumer-social movements (see Chapter 2), dominant professional models or paradigms (see Chapters 2 and 6), and professionalization. Nevertheless, reprofessionalization with concomitant attitudinal, knowledge, and role changes can be considered congruent with the premises of primary health care that assumes reliance on lay health workers (World Health Organization, 1978) and partnership with laypersons. Clearly the principal obstacle to appropriate professional relationships with consumers and their social networks is the nexus of attitudes and values that underlie professionalism as an ideology. To the extent that this ideology—and these attitudes and values—characterizes all professions, including nursing, it would seem that the educational means of combating that ideology should be applicable to nursing, too.

Relevant Learning Opportunities

Nurse educators can glean some guidance from the few pertinent programs in other health professions. At the University of Toronto in Canada, medical students meet in seminars with members of self-help groups (Kelner, 1986) in a program that stresses experiential strategies (Romeder, 1982). Two European medical schools have sponsored seminars on self-help groups (Branckaerts, 1983). Bremer-Schulte

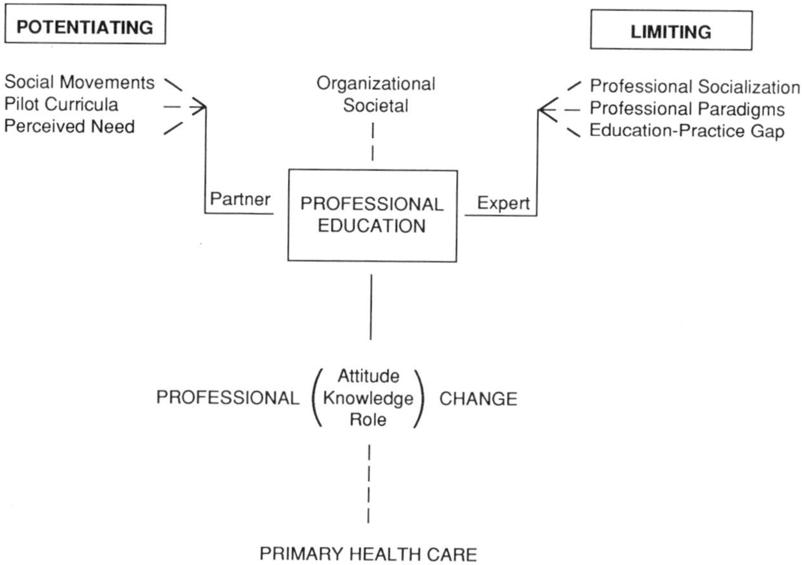

Figure 7.1. Factors Influencing Effectiveness of Professional Education to Prepare for Work With Lay Groups

(1983) describes how medical education can be aimed at attitude development to stimulate and facilitate self-care and self-help. One curriculum for social workers seeks initially to "undermine students' trust and beliefs in the ascendance of technology and force a re-examination of a professional enterprise that casts nonprofessionals into the subservient role of client," through experiential and didactic elements (Gottlieb & Farquharson, 1985). The emphasis on experiential teaching strategies in these reported programs may be derived not only from a grounding in educational theory but also from efforts to be congruent with the experiential knowledge core of self-help groups; however, this is never explicitly stated.

Clearly the educational preparation of some health professionals for work with self-help groups has barely begun. Complex challenges lie ahead and widespread implementation is needed. Although the impact of these curricula and programs has not been empirically evaluated, gaps are discernible. For example, consultation skills, significant for symmetrical interaction with consumers, do not appear to be stressed in these curricula. Lenrow and Burch (1981) hope that interdependence of professionals with clients will become a principle modeled in professional education and exemplified in professional practice. Correspondingly, Borkman (1990) refers to the egalitarian alliances emerging between self-help groups and the formal health-care system. However, Katz (1985) recommends that "as long as it (interdependence) remains an unrealized vision . . . emphasis in professional curricula . . . on self-help forms should occur" (p. 134). This has implications for classroom and clinical learning opportunities for nursing students and for the conceptual framework on which these opportunities are based.

Classroom Focus for Nursing Students

All educational offerings should stress knowledge of social support premises and of the prospects and problems of professional partnership with laypersons. In classroom and tutorial settings, selected content foci could include:

1. Premises and principles of primary health care
2. The relevance of social (lay) support to health professionals and nurses (i.e., impact on health, on health behavior, and on health-services utilization)
3. The commonalities and distinctions between professional and lay helpers
4. Major theoretical viewpoints concerning social support
5. Theories relevant to social support (including mutual aid) with concrete examples
6. Theoretical and empirical contributions of nurses to the social support knowledge base
7. Comparison of nursing surrogate support and lay support
8. Appropriate nursing roles vis-à-vis informal helpers (individuals/groups/networks) and individual clients

In tutorial sessions, students can be guided to examine their own experiences with informal helping, as Gottlieb and Farquharson (1985) prescribe. For example, nurse learners could map their own social support networks and view videotapes of a self-help/mutual-aid interchange. Group experiences in tutorials/seminars should help these students to develop skills for use with self-help groups. Finally, the self-help/consumerism movement suggests specific types of teaching/learning strategies such as student debates that, like social movements, encourage confrontation and challenge. Thus experiential knowledge is evoked.

Clinical Focus for Nursing Students

Experiential learning opportunities also can be expanded through field assignments and clinical placements. These opportunities should prepare student nurses for assuming primary health care roles in a variety of sites. Role modeling by faculty and by other student nurses and role playing can facilitate this process. "Reflection-in-action"—a term coined by Schon (1987)—and critical analysis by students could be emphasized didactically and experientially. Case studies and small-group discussions could elicit pertinent life experiences. Group experiences in tutorials/seminars should help nursing students develop skills for use with self-help and support groups. Such skills include facilitation, rather than leadership, of group interactions and community or group development and empowerment. Thus students would learn to guide rather than co-opt groups.

The clinical focus would be on preparing nurses to work in enabling, consultative, and partner roles rather than traditional expert-caregiver roles. This assumes empowerment of consumers at collective levels and promotion of individual consumer self-efficacy. Thus student nurses would learn how to mobilize and enhance informal helping by natural and created networks. Faculty would need to ensure that opportunities for facilitating lay networks, mutual-aid groups, neighborhood helpers, volunteer linkage, and community empowerment were included as appropriate within clinical experiences. Specific attention in curricula would be given to developing referral, linkage, teaching, consultant, helper, and partner roles. (These roles were introduced in Chapter 4 and defined in Chapter 6.) Thus nursing students would discern that assistance should be temporary; should result in enhanced opportunity and self-actualization for the consumer; and can come not only from themselves but also from clients, clients' social network, and clients' peers. This is in direct contrast to the traditional medical model (discussed in Chapter 2) and reflects partnership.

Collaborative partnership roles can be mastered when there is negotiation among nursing students, clients, and lay helpers regarding respective goals, responsibilities, role expectations, and status in interactions. The student can, through consultation, facilitate resocialization of laypersons and support networks from traditional, passive role expectations to new partner roles. Hence equality in levels of status, control, and responsibility would ensue.

Learned interventions could focus on mobilization of support from key network members, introduction of new supportive ties, optimizing support rendered by the existing network, grafting on a set of new ties, and public educational strategies. Thus nursing students could facilitate creation of self-help groups for parents of hospitalized children or could link pairs of hospitalized children with the same condition and approximately the same age. Similarly, student nurses can encourage elderly residents to lobby for development of such supportive environments as senior citizen apartments, buddy systems, supportive neighbors who daily visit or contact each other, and volunteer services such as Friendly Visitors or foster grandparents (Stewart, 1988). Other potential target groups with which students might have contact are childbearing couples, new parents, the chronically ill, the bereaved, caregivers of dependent family members, or victims of abuse. For example, nursing students taught prenatal classes to adolescent single mothers, and observed reciprocity within these support groups (Wuest, 1990). (See Chapter 4 for exemplified interventions.) Skill development would emphasize consultation skills, group work skills, community organization skills, and leadership skills. Experiential assignments for professional-role development in relation to support groups, as one example of social support, are outlined in Table 7.1.

Adapted Conceptual Framework for Nursing Curriculum

Some studies reveal that the environment (society) appears less frequently than the other three metaparadigm concepts in conceptual frameworks of nursing curricula. For example, King (1986) found that the use of environmental terms such as *social system* is inconsistent. The environment domain, as noted in the preceding chapter, also has been neglected in nursing practice models. A new framework, based on the theoretical framework proposed in Chapter 6, could contribute to nursing education by conceptually explicating the environment. In

Table 7.1 Experiential Learning Opportunities

1. Conduct community needs assessment to determine available services and service gaps around which mutual-aid groups might be developed
2. Observe support group meetings and describe group dynamics and group members' roles
3. Perform case studies of existing groups
4. Make oral presentation on activities associated with self-help groups
5. Distinguish professional intervention from lay helping patterns
6. Use community organization concepts and skills to identify natural resources and to develop/maintain self-help groups
7. Assess current self-help groups and models
8. Identify and develop list of self-help groups in the community
9. Identify tensions between professional and informal (lay) health services and prospects for partnership
10. Describe roles played by professionals at various stages of development of self-help groups
11. Assess organizational settings for possible introduction of self-help groups
12. Spot and encourage leadership in self-help groups
13. Conduct public opinion surveys regarding necessity for self-help groups and other support interventions
14. Germinate self-help groups with agency or clinic and transplant them in community
15. Videotape actual self-help group interactions using guidelines to examine group dynamics

Adapted from Gottlieb & Farquharson, 1985.

fact, Sword, Noesgaard, and Majumdar (1992) applied this model to baccalaureate nursing students' learning experiences in nontraditional community settings. The holistic environment and the nurse-person partnership were confirmed.

The assumptions for a social support framework for a nursing curriculum would emphasize professional collaboration with laypersons and lay helping networks. They would reflect premises concerning the nature of human beings, their environments, health and health care, and nursing that are consistent with a social rather than a medical model perspective. For example:

> Human beings have the right to independent choice and control with respect to help from their social environments and from student nurses. Primary health care by student nurses and social support from environments each encompass lay helping.

Furthermore, conceptualization of the role of the nurse would emphasize a move toward consultant, partner, and primary health care roles, rather than institutionalized care of ill individuals primarily. The *primary health care role* could be defined as follows: The primary health care role, assumed by the student nurse, requires mutual cooperation with clients and with social network members to enhance access to combined lay/professional services and thus to promote health of clients.

A sample relationship statement follows:

> Reciprocal exchange of information derived from the student nurse's professional knowledge, the client's experiential knowledge, and the social network's experiential knowledge should promote partnership role assumption by each party.

These examples are directly derived from the theoretical framework advanced in Chapter 6, which can be modified for both education and practice. According to Tilden (1985b), "At this date enough research and theory development has occurred to assure the place of social support as a major construct in nursing science . . . educational curricula may be increasingly focused on this concept" (p. 13). This adapted conceptual framework for nursing education based on social support could provide useful guidelines for this important development. Teaching and learning theories also are important ingredients of undergraduate nursing-school frameworks.

Health-professional curricula are influenced by internal, intraorganizational, and external societal forces, which interact to create a professional preparation environment that in turn influences the design of educational processes intended to achieve professional-preparation outcomes (Stark et al., 1986). Consequently, "revolutionary" thinkers in the human-service fields, both health (Wright & Treacher, 1982) and education (Popkewitz, 1984), emphasize "social practice" and linkage with society rather than the traditional view of distinctive spheres. This implies that nurses need to acknowledge and interact with informal social networks. Hence nursing curricular changes must reflect an understanding of the reproductive dimensions in a society that make orientations resistant to change. The "lived experience" of nursing students will act as a mediating force in what is actually taught, learned, and rejected.

Nurse educators and theorists teach and write about nursing "as it ought to be," while practicing nurses perceive nursing "as it is" within the multiple constraints of the institutional system (Benner, 1984). Therefore nurses contemplating change should preserve the idealism that is necessary if they are to prepare for the challenge of consumer-support movements and appropriate roles, but temper that idealism with realism. It is to be hoped that nurse preparation for appropriate partner roles through educational programs will in the long term enhance lay networks and expedite consumer education. Clearly, relevant progressive curricula are needed to prepare nurses to meet changing societal needs.

Social Support for Students and Faculty

Social support is significant not only for nursing clientele but also for nurses themselves. Recently, the impact of support on health-professional students and educators has received some attention. Self-help groups have proven effective in mitigating the stress experienced by professional nurses and by students from other disciplines. For example, medical students who participate in self-help groups themselves report benefits such as amelioration of loneliness, support from peers, and insight into problem solving (Goetzel et al., 1983). Ihlenfield (1991) describes how nursing students retained friendship only with peers who provided support in student nurse clinical groups. Lack of peer support and conflicted support were predictors of nursing student attrition (Marshall, 1989). Social support was positively related to the evaluation of challenge, in student appraisal of stress, in an initial clinical nursing situation (Pagana, 1990). Vance (1990) contends that mentors and other supporters are essential for developing professionals. For these reasons, self-help groups and other support mechanisms could be created for nursing students.

Chapters 4 and 5 appraise the value of occupational support for practicing nurses. Faculty also require this type of support. Fong (1990) reported that the degree of support from supervisors and peers correlated significantly and negatively with burnout of nursing educators. Lack of peer support predicted depersonalization toward students, and chairperson support predicted sense of accomplishment. Clearly, social support strategies also could be instigated for nurse educators.

Summary

Nurses and other health professionals report deficiencies in their knowledge and skill base pertaining to social support groups and lay helpers. Modification in attitudes and roles, consistent with the shift from a medical model orientation to a social model, is propitious. Reprofessionalization for pertinent practice competencies, attitudes, and knowledge can be achieved in part through formal education of nurses. Premises of social support and its significance for nursing can be conveyed in classroom and clinical settings, particularly if incorporated in the curriculum's conceptual framework. However, divergent organizational and societal forces will influence the impact of progressive curricula that are grounded on social support premises. Likewise, the relevance of support to the stress encountered by nursing educators and students will influence the preparation of nurses for the transition from provider to partner.

❖ CHAPTER EIGHT ❖

Projection and Prospectus

Clearly social support is salient to nursing practice, research, theory, and education. Nurses play important indirect and direct support roles with varied target populations in sundry sites. Furthermore, nurses have contributed to the conceptualization, measurement, and empirical study of social support and its relationship to the health of diverse populations. Some groundwork has been laid in overcoming nurses' knowledge and skill deficiencies pertaining to work with lay helpers and networks of clientele and in preparing nurses for appropriate partnership roles. Nevertheless, some obstacles and gaps persist that suggest directions for future efforts by nurse researchers, theoreticians, practitioners, and educators to advance and apply the study of social support. A prospectus for this nursing work is proposed in this chapter.

Conceptual Controversies

The call for precise concepts and models continues. Nurses can contribute to enhanced theoretical interpretations of the operating mechanisms and component processes of support and of support's linkage to health. Debate continues surrounding the dimensionality of support and functional versus structural approaches to analyzing support. Drawbacks of support, which influence providers' and recipients' functioning, self-esteem, and health, require further attention. There has been insufficient research about the negative effects of social networks, and measures of support typically disregard the negative aspects of relationships. Theoreticians, researchers, and practitioners should take into account both negative and positive features of social interactions—interpersonal stress and interpersonal support. The reciprocal relationship between coping strategies (which reduce or manage stress) and social support requires further conceptualization and testing.

Theoretical grounding of the empirical studies conducted and instruments created by nurses is not widespread. A few researchers logically invoke coping-stress theory. Alternatively, reciprocity, social learning, social competence, and social comparison theories may need to be applied for logical congruency. As noted in Chapter 5, only one instrument was based on equity theory. Regrettably no intervention studies were theoretically based, despite the espoused need for support intervention trials with theoretical frameworks. Only four nursing studies tested or developed models that link social support to health status, health practices, coping effectiveness, or caring. Furthermore, only one nursing report explicitly linked social support theory and nursing theory, an important but limited achievement, as consumers and lay networks are rarely represented in nursing theories. Nurses have generated but not tested other models to elucidate the construct of social support. In fact, Norbeck (1988b) contends that social support theory development could guide nursing practice. Accordingly, a nursing conceptual model derived from social support theories, such as the one proposed in Chapter 6, may be timely.

Two conceptual controversies that could be clarified by the future work of nurses are the negative features of interactions and social relationships, and the linkages among stress, coping, support, and health.

Negative Features of Interactions and Social Relationships

The quality of specific types and sources of support may vary greatly along a continuum from positive to negative, depending on the interaction, situation, or relationship. Reports of low support may reflect the absence of a supportive relationship or the presence of a negative, conflicted relationship (Coyne & Bolger, 1990) or lost support (Robinson, 1990). Conflict, inhibited communication, negative interactions, and lack of stability correlate more strongly than positive interactions with decreased perceived support and increased psychological symptoms (Coyne & Downey, 1991; Schuster et al., 1990). Linkages of negative and positive features of social relationships with psychological and physical health states require further conceptualization and testing by nurses and other disciplines. For example, the costs of social ties for children and adolescents, in the form of negative interpersonal exchanges and stressful events in network members' lives, have not been analyzed (Compas, 1991), although attachment theory suggests the impact of the loss of supportive others. Conversely, individual characteristics may alter the quality and quantity of support sought and received. People who exhibit hostile behavior may perceive interactions intended to be supportive as nonsupportive, may alienate others, or may avoid seeking support (Houston & Vavak, 1991). Hence the quality of personal and social factors influencing support should be elucidated.

Both the supportive and nonsupportive features of interactions and relationships should be assessed concurrently by nurses. The positive and negative impact of confidants and family members, such as siblings and grandparents (Clements et al., 1990), is not clearly understood. Underuse and overuse of resources can be interpreted by reciprocity and self-esteem theory (Fisher et al., 1988), and support interventions by nurses can alleviate disparate views.

Equity theory enables interpretation of some negative features of relationships and of how providing support (e.g., caregiving) drains resources. Rook (1987) and Tilburg, Sonderen, and Ormel (1991) distinguish four operationalizations of reciprocity—"total"/summated, additivity in relationships, relationship-specific, and support (type)-specific. However, a match between giving and receiving may not be required (Antonucci & Israel, 1986). A theoretical interpretation of the link between reciprocity and psychosocial well-being is lacking (Tilburg et al., 1991). The long-term nature of the reciprocity of resources in ongoing relationships of kin and intimates should be recognized and reinforced by nurses. Furthermore, inequitable relationships that may result from illness, aging, and interactions with health professionals should be minimized.

Theoretical formulations and techniques of assessing support have not yet come to terms with the fact that negative features of relationships predominate in influencing support perceptions (Coyne &

Downey, 1991). A multidimensional conceptualization of negative social interactions may be useful.

Stress, Coping, Support, and Health Linkages

"Social support is as much a complex process of accommodation to the needs of close relationships as it is an accommodation to stress" (Gottlieb & Wagner, 1991). The means by which involvement in dysfunctional relationships impairs coping with stress require study (Coyne & Downey, 1991). Specific stressors and burden types require greater explication. Coyne, Ellard, and Smith (1990) observe that "simple correlations among measures of stress, support and adaptational outcomes . . . tell us little about the circumstances producing these associations" (p. 131). Therefore, conceptualization of "relationship-focused" coping could supplement the traditional study of emotion- and problem-focused coping (Coyne & Downey, 1991).

The bidirectional relationship between social support and health has not been fully conceptualized; there has been more attention to the impact of support on health than to the impact of health status on support received and sought. Hence there is a need to test the conceptual processes by which support influences health, both in the presence of and irrespective of coping and stress. Longitudinal studies should facilitate this effort. Certainly new frameworks, created or modified by nurses, may help to interpret the positive and negative features of support and the mechanisms by which support works and interacts with health.

Design Dilemmas

Regrettably, extant measures do not reflect the multifaceted nature of the construct, process, or interaction and communication of support. Measures should distinguish positive and negative interactions. Measures for different ethnic groups or cultures are virtually nonexistent, despite Norbeck and Tilden's (1988) assertion of the need to test whether social support is a universal construct. There has been insufficient psychometric testing of social support instruments or attention to construct validity by nurses. To overcome proliferation of nursing instruments, repeated application of a few measures to different target populations is propitious. For example, nurses could use measures specifically designed for children, such as those recognized by Gottlieb and Selby (1989). Nurses, however, have begun to develop situation- and population-specific measures, which should make possible the specific matching of measurements of stressors, support, and well-being, as is recommended in the social-psychological literature.

Social support research by nurses is predominantly cross-sectional and quantitative. Longitudinal studies are needed to reveal the causal process through which support influences health and, conversely, health status influences support; to divulge the mechanisms of support; to follow at-risk populations (e.g., isolated, ill, bereaved, elderly, persons with undeveloped social competence); and to evaluate the effects of support interventions over time. The aim of nursing research and selected dimensions of nursing measures should be, as Norbeck (1988b) recommends, to add to the predictive power of social support-stress-health models. Conspicuous cross-sectional designs and deficient quantitative measures lead to speculation that the critical process and mechanisms of support may be uncovered not only by longitudinal research but also by qualitative and participatory research designs.

Longitudinal Design

Prospective, longitudinal studies are needed to reflect a life-course development perspective of the influences of social support on men's and women's health over time (Coyne & Downey, 1991; Rodin & Ickovics, 1990; Shumaker & Hill, 1991). Prospective research could reveal how the sources and nature of support may change with age (Compas, 1991) and could test the stress-moderator effects of support following life events (Blaney et al., 1991). Furthermore, reciprocity in continuing close relationships can be interpreted for different age groups (Tilburg et al., 1991). Frequently, studies have operationalized social networks without consideration of age, and those that have taken age into account (e.g., Olson, Ivarson, & Sabree, 1991) unfortunately have not employed longitudinal designs. Furthermore, many projects have inappropriately applied definitions of support developed for adult populations to children and adolescents (Compas, 1991). Thus longitudinal designs, if intrinsic in nursing research, can explicate the support process, enable evaluation of the direction of support's relationship with health, and reflect the evolution of individuals and relationships.

Qualitative Design

Qualitative research is consistent with comprehending experiential phenomena such as support and its changes over time (Powell & Cameron, 1991), yet has rarely been conducted by nurse investigators. Experimental and quantitative designs, although capable of testing effects and interactions, may not capture the transactional complexity of support and the support process. Semistructured, qualitative interviews can interpret theoretical relationships between support and health (Coyne & Downey, 1991; Heller, 1990). There is a risk that imposing the rigor of quantitative design on natural networks and support groups may change their nature (Goldklang, 1991). In qualitative designs, theoretical or purposive sampling is consistent with the theoretical requirements of the research. Reliability can be ensured by checking information and themes with secondary informants. Validity can be achieved by selecting exceptions or negative cases (Morse, 1989). Nevertheless, debates among nurses concerning the rigor of qualitative versus quantitative designs persist.

Audio- and videotape recordings and communication rating scales are available (Garvin & Kennedy, 1990) for qualitative data. Content analysis is one type of qualitative research analytic technique; others include analytic induction, semiotics, hermeneutics, discourse analysis, and grounded theory. These approaches are appropriate when little is known about a phenomenon or when what is known is suspected to be biased, and the purpose of the study is to describe the phenomenon from the perspective of the person who is experiencing it (Field & Morse, 1985; Kirk & Miller, 1986; Potter & Wetherell, 1989).

Clearly there are increasing calls for attention to the study of the process of supportive interactions among self-help group members (e.g., Maton, 1988; Powell & Cameron, 1991) and in close personal relationships (e.g., Gottlieb & Wagner, 1991). For example, an otherwise well-designed randomized control trial of a telephone support intervention for socioeconomically disadvantaged women (Heller, Thompson, Trueba, Hogg, & Vlachos-Weber, 1991) was criticized for its inattention to process (e.g., Gottlieb, 1991). Recognition of process-focused research as much as outcome-oriented study is needed (Goldklang, 1991). Accordingly, the status of qualitative research, elevated recently by nurse methodologists, could be acknowledged by nurse investigators focusing on social support.

Participatory Research

Participatory and applied research share certain characteristics germane to nursing research on social support. Subjects are engaged as active participants in order to consider their assumptions and social situations (similar to ethnographic qualitative research). Ongoing communication, training, and joint decision making throughout problem identification, planning, intervention, and evaluation are critical (LeBoterf, 1983; Maclure, 1991; Ramphele, 1990). Focus groups, workshops, and interviews can be selected as strategies (Goldklang, 1991).

Chesler (1991) contrasts conventional research, in which researchers are detached, objective, and in control, with participatory research, where there is co-control or even participant (subject) control. Barriers to participatory research are created by researchers' preference for traditional quantitative methods and by the conflicting views of participants and researchers (Powell & Cameron, 1991). The "participatory" paradigm is congruent with research pertaining to self-help groups and lay helpers because it values equity, empowerment, learned skills, developmental changes, social processes (Brown & Tandon, 1983; Chesler, 1991; Powell & Cameron, 1991), and the legitimization and creation of new social roles for participants of support interventions (Stein, 1991). A compromise between the long-term significance of basic research and the short-term usefulness of applied research may be necessary. The premises of shared ownership, learning, and action reveal that participatory research is one mode of applied research very relevant to support interventions by nurses.

Practice Priorities

Intervention field trials by nurses should be applied to nursing practice. Many intervention studies by nurses have encompassed professional support only. Although the four that entailed lay support were longitudinal, only two had a randomized control trial design (Chapter 5). There is a need for controlled intervention trials based on theory. The positive and negative impact of interventions should be documented. All levels of intervention should be evaluated in terms of their impact on outcomes, their mixed effects, their side effects, their maintenance over time, and their long-term effects. Furthermore, intervention processes need to be clearly delineated. Nurse researchers have focused more on the buffering than the main effects of support on health, and on psychological rather than physical health outcomes. Studies of the impact of primary prevention interventions on health behavior, positive health outcomes, well-being, life satisfaction, and functioning are therefore needed. (For example, social competence interventions for the lonely may optimize support receipt and self-esteem.) There have been few measures of effectiveness or outcomes in nursing reports of support groups and no interventions that entailed community forums or social systems.

Professional-role redefinition to enable help seeking from lay sources and enhance relevance to consumer needs (representing a shift in paradigms and influences of social movements) exemplifies social system-level interventions. Deficiencies in nurse preparation for partner roles and for interactions with lay networks of clients point to the need to enhance nursing and consumer education (Chapter 7). Professional socialization may have to be altered to instill attitudes and values that reflect new, holistic, social-health paradigms.

Interventions should be matched to needs. There is a need to address gaps in nursing research, and perhaps practice, in terms of children and members of lower socioeconomic groups or non-dominant cultures. Women also have been neglected in social support studies, despite the marked differences in their needs, provision and impact of support, and social relationships with respect to those of men. Nursing, as a predominantly female profession, can contribute to the understanding of gender in social support research and interventions.

Interventions

Interventions can modify or mobilize natural networks, create new sources of support, decrease conflict, or enhance the quality of support in close personal relationships (Barrera, 1991; Maguire, 1991; Vaux, 1989). The context of personal relationships (Stein, 1991) and "the supportive dimension of participants' commerce with their social fields, including their wants and needs for support" (Gottlieb, 1991, p. 124) should be assessed prior to designing interventions. Interventions designed to strengthen social resources can occur at community, organizational, interpersonal, and individual levels (Heller, 1990). Thus classroom and work settings may be just as suitable sites for nursing-support interventions as are home and hospital.

Support interventions are most useful when they restore or enhance role functioning, reinforce existing social structures, develop new skills, enable coping with stressful transitions (Heller, 1990; Thoits, 1986), or alleviate social isolation and feelings of loss (Maguire, 1991). For example, family caregiver techniques could be taught by nurses (Lindeman, 1988). Such interventions can moderate the costs of providing and seeking support that are associated with overuse and underuse of resources (Fisher et al., 1988) from specific sources.

One type of intervention that has engendered increasing interest among other disciplines, and which that be applied and developed by nurses, is telephone support. Thus low-technology, low-cost programs can link elderly persons who live alone (King, 1991), children (Kliewer, Lepore, Broquet, & Zuba, 1990; Peterson, 1990), people with AIDS (Rounds, Galinsky, & Stevens, 1991), or other groups living in rural communities by communicating support of peers and professionals. Heller, Thompson, Trueba, Hogg, & Vlachos-Weber (1991) tested a preventive intervention of peer telephone dyads for low-income elderly women with low perceived support; however, it was unclear whether improved mental-health status could be attributed to the support intervention or to participation in the study.

Therefore, support intervention programs should be followed by close periodic assessment of physical or psychosocial health status (Florian & Krulik, 1991) or other positive health or functioning indicators. Thus parenting and work effectiveness might be as appropriate outcomes of nursing interventions as positive or negative health status. Surrogate support by nurses (Swanson, 1991) also should be tested for its impact on health status. Longitudinal studies may have unintended intervention effects, such as those reported in a nursing study of family caregivers who appraised their experience relative to that of other caregivers, altered problem-solving strategies, and sought additional support (Collins, Given, & Berry, 1989). Group interventions may need to be lengthier and to have better measures of psychological variables to demonstrate the relationship between improved coping, reduced stress, and improved mental health (Toseland et al., 1989). Furthermore, comparative studies are needed to examine the differences between the support and coping behaviors of people who belong to mutual-aid groups and those of people who do not (Rheume & Gooding, 1991) and to document the long- and short-term outcomes of group participation in terms of coping and family dynamics (Betz et al., 1990). Educational interventions (Lindeman, 1988), combined with support, require further testing. Clearly nurses need training in support interventions and in evaluation of intervention outcomes and processes.

Gender

Although investigations of the links between women's support and health are rare, women have an advantage over men with respect to mortality, and low social support has been linked to increased risk of morbidity (Rodin & Ickovics, 1990; Shumaker & Hill, 1991). The weaker, more complex, relationship between physical health and social support for women may relate to the fact that women have more confidants throughout their life span, their networks are more multifaceted, and they are more likely to give all types of support and to mobilize their support networks (Belle, 1987; Flaherty & Richman, 1989). Psychological and social variables (such as social support, poverty, perceived control, life roles, and redefined gender roles) influence women's health (Maguire, 1991; Rodin & Ickovics, 1990). Involvement in multiple roles, for example, expands women's potential support resources and self-esteem, which in turn enhances their mental and physical health (Sorensen & Verbrugge, 1987).

Gender differences in coping responses to a common stressor were revealed in Gottlieb and Wagner's (1991) qualitative study of the parents of a child with a chronic illness, which in turn engendered conflict in these close personal relationships. Reciprocity in relationships influences women's, more than men's, support satisfaction (Antonucci & Akijama, 1987). Furthermore, women tend to be exposed more to negative social interactions and outcomes, perhaps due to increased caregiving roles, yet benefit more from supportive interactions (Schuster et al., 1990; Shumaker & Hill, 1991). These distinctions in support seeking, provision, and outcomes should be illuminated in nursing research and reflected in nursing interventions.

Partnership

The women's movement exemplifies critical consumer movements. Educated consumers and a true partnership between consumers and providers could markedly influence health care and health policy (Rehr & Rosenberg, 1991). The balance theory of coordination was applied by Kurtz (1990) to analyze balanced involvement, underinvolvement, and overinvolvement of professionals with mutual-aid groups. Concerns regarding the impact of professionals on the autonomy and authenticity of groups (Powell & Cameron, 1991) and diffusion of the reform orientation of these manifestations of social movements (Emerick, 1991) reflect overinvolvement. Qualitative and quantitative designs measuring process and outcomes of these different levels of relationships between nurses and laypersons are therefore needed.

Potential conflicts, however, also may exist between the natural social network and outside peer resources—nurses could then recommend the use of other lay or professional sources of support. Clearly education of nurses for pertinent interventions and partnership roles is essential. Educational strategies such as those proposed in Chapter 7 are timely.

Concluding Comments

Nurses have made significant strides in the scrutiny and manipulation of social support from practice, research, theory, and education perspectives. Nevertheless, persisting controversies and oversights require resolution.

The negative and positive features of social interactions and relationships, and the interaction of support and health, can be elucidated by nurse theoreticians and investigators, and guide nursing interventions. Qualitative and longitudinal designs can uncover pertinent processes and mechanisms of support.

Qualitative and participatory research strategies also are consistent with the feminist and cultural perspectives that typically have been overlooked. Furthermore, participatory research is consonant with future educational preparation of nurses for partnership in practice. Clearly social support will continue to have significance for nursing.

Commentary

In the course of science, concepts and their surrounding theories occasionally emerge that are so salient to a discipline that knowledge in that discipline is forever altered. Social support is such a concept. Long before the concept of social support made its debut in the late 1960s as a health variable, nurses and nursing embodied and enacted social support within their domain of knowledge and practice. However, it was not until the pioneering, seminal ideas of Gerald Caplan, John Cassel, and Sidney Cobb that health scientists, including nurse scientists, sought to systematically study the links between human support and health outcomes.

Nursing science takes a broad view of the client in the context of his or her environment, especially the client's interpersonal environment. Thus social support and its attending theories are pivotal to nurses. There are at least three reasons that knowledge of social support is significant for the science of nursing. First, recent health-care trends, especially those related to the financing of health care, have made social networks central to health-care delivery. Health-care demographics mean that families must shoulder much of the responsibility for care of patients, who now have brief hospital stays, live longer, and have far more chronic, long-term conditions than ever before in history. Knowledge of social support allows nurses to facilitate the ability of families and the wider social network to be more successful and adaptive caregivers—with less burden, burnout, and negative health sequelae of their own.

Second, the consumer revolution brought the self-help movement into center stage of the health-care arena. Tired of a paternalistic, hierarchical health-care system that traditionally has eschewed experiential knowledge, consumers now demand a partnership with providers and recognition for their contributions. Self-help/mutual-aid groups now exist for every conceivable health-related condition. Such groups are really an extension of social networks, and they provide supplies of emotional, affirmational, informational, and tangible support. Nurses collaborate with self-help groups in important ways as program planners, consultants, evaluators, and sources of referral.

Third, the health-care delivery system has become more health promotive and disease preventive than ever before in history; the greater benefits of preventing illness as opposed to treating illness are obvious. Research evidence indicates that social support acts to buffer stress and lessen morbidity and mortality, and nurses use this knowledge in their primary and secondary prevention programs.

Nurses have contributed substantively to the now 30 years of research and theory development about social support, and they deserve a large amount of the credit for what is known about this concept today. Thus it is timely and appropriate that a nurse scientist gives us this synthesizing text that stands as a testament to nursing's contribution to social support knowledge development.

In this book, Dr. Stewart draws together the vast literature about this illusive concept, and lights the path through the maze of definitions, explanatory theories, conceptual models, measures, and study findings. In the early chapters, she describes the diverse definitions and theoretical interpretations of the concept, its hypothesized mechanisms of action, its costs and benefits, and the self-help movement that bridged informal, unorganized helping relationships and formal, professional care. Against this backdrop, familiar to students of the concept, Stewart then breaks new ground by focusing on the significance of social support to nursing science; the contributions of nurses to social support knowledge development; and the role of nurses as they intervene with social support inoculations at individual, dyadic, and group levels. Although other nurse authors have written on the topic, this is the first text on social support in nursing and the first text that puts nursing center stage as an applied discipline using descriptive knowledge about this concept to effect change.

Stewart concludes by beaming the light on future directions. Science of the concept is far from complete, and the author chronicles for us the most urgent needs: better measures to replace those Norbeck has called "first generation" instruments, more intervention studies with measurable and significant outcomes, more clarity about why gender is such a strong predictor of social support and why social support seems to function differently for women and men, and more clarity about the stress-producing components of support relationships.

Although much lies ahead to accomplish in scientific investigation of the concept, this book suggests an emerging approach to our educational programs, based on social support, that views clients/patients as partners and families as allies. This approach values the patient's and family's knowledge and experience and includes their world view in the treatment plan. To this I add three closing challenges.

First, in your clinical practice, avoid vague and weak language. Nursing has overused the phrases "assess social support" and "provide support to the patient." Use this book to operationalize your meaning. If you say your practice includes assessment of the social network prior to discharge of a patient, state exactly what you will assess: size? frequency of contact? degree of conflict? density? satisfaction? perceived available support? If you determine a social support deficit or dysfunction, be specific about its indicators and, if appropriate, your planned intervention.

Second, if you plan to measure social support in your research, select a measure to operationalize the concept that is congruent with your conception of the concept. Also, select a measure for which published psychometric information exists, so your future publications contribute to the science of the concept and its measurement through comparability of findings and validity assessment of the measure. We perpetuate weak science when we choose measures that are incongruent with the conception of the study or those without evidence of reliability and validity.

Third, apply knowledge of social support to your own work environment. Why is it that nurses are so much better at prescribing support for patients while allowing our own professional relationships to be isolative, competitive, and nonaffirming? We can use the concept, which we know to be health promotive for our patients, to alter our work communities, thereby bringing to ourselves the benefits of this rich and enduring human glue called social support.

Virginia Tilden, M.D.

References

Aaronson, L. S. (1989). Perceived and received support: Effects on health behaviour during pregnancy. *Nursing Research, 38*(1), 4-9.

Abood, D. A., & Milton, S. (1988). A path analytic model for investigating the relationship among stress, illness, social support, and health practices. *Health Education, 19*(4), 22-26.

Adams, J. S. (1963). Toward an understanding of inequity. *Journal of Abnormal and Social Psychology, 67*, 422-436.

Adelman, M., Parks, M., & Albrecht, T. (1987). Supporting friends in need. In T. Albrecht & M. Adelman (Eds.), *Communicating social support* (pp. 62-75). Newbury Park, CA: Sage.

Ahmadi, K. S. (1985). The experience of being hospitalized: Stress, social support and satisfaction. *International Journal of Nursing Studies, 22*, 137-148.

Albrecht, S. A., & Rankin, M. (1989). Anxiety levels, health behaviors, and support-systems of pregnant women. *Maternal-Child Nursing Journal, 18*(1), 49-60.

Albrecht, T., & Adelman, M. (1987). Communication networks as structures of social support. In T. Albrecht & M. Adelman (Eds.), *Communicating social support* (pp. 40-61). Newbury Park, CA: Sage.

Allender, J. S. (1986). Educational research: A personal and social process. *Review of Educational Research, 56*, 173-193.

Alley, N., & Foster, M. (1990). Using self-help support groups: A framework for nursing practice and research. *Journal of Advanced Nursing, 15*, 1383-1388.

Anderson, J. L. (1989). The nurse's role in cancer rehabilitation. *Cancer Nursing, 12*(2), 85-93.

Anderson, J. M., & Elfert, H. (1989). Managing chronic illness in the family: Women as caretakers. *Journal of Advanced Nursing, 14*, 735-743.

Antonucci, T. C. (1985). Social support: Theoretical advances, recent findings and pressing issues. In I. G. Sarason & B. R. Sarason (Eds.), *Social support: Theory, research, application* (pp. 21-37). Dordrecht, The Netherlands: Martinus Nijhoff.

Antonucci, T. C., & Akiyama, H. (1987). An examination of sex differences in social support in mid and late life. *Sex Roles, 17*, 737-749.

Antonucci, T. C., & Depner, C. E. (1982). Social support and informal helping relationships. In T. A. Wills (Ed.), *Basic processes in helping relationships* (pp. 233-254). New York: Academic Press.

Antonucci, T. C., & Israel, B. (1986). Veridicality of social support: A comparison of principal and network members' responses. *Journal of Consulting and Clinical Psychology, 54,* 432-437.

Antonucci, T. C., & Jackson, J. S. (1990). The role of reciprocity in social support. In B. R. Sarason, I. G. Sarason, & G. R. Pierce (Eds.), *Social support: An interactional view* (pp. 173-198). New York: John Wiley.

Apple, M., & Weiss, L. (1983). *Ideology and practice in schooling.* Philadelphia: Temple University Press.

Auslander, G., & Litwin, H. (1990). Social support networks and formal help seeking: Differences between applicants to social services and a non-applicant sample. *Journal of Gerontology, 45*(3), 5112-5119.

Baillie, V., Norbeck, J., & Barnes, L. (1988). Stress, social support and psychological distress of family caregivers of the elderly. *Nursing Research, 37*(4), 217-222.

Bandura, A. (1977). Self-efficacy: Toward a unifying theory of behavioral change. *Psychological Review, 84*(2), 191-215.

Bandura, A. (1986). *A social foundation of thought and action: A social cognitive theory.* Englewood Cliffs, NJ: Prentice Hall.

Bandura, A., Reese, L., & Adams, N. (1982). Microanalysis of action and fear arousal as a function of differential levels of perceived self-efficacy. *Journal of Personality and Social Psychology, 43*(1), 5-21.

Banks, S. (1985). *Informal learning in self-help groups.* Unpublished master's thesis, Dalhousie University, Halifax, Nova Scotia, Canada.

Barbarin, O. A., & Chesler, M. (1986). The medical context of parental coping with childhood cancer. *American Journal of Community Psychology, 14*(2), 221-235.

Barbee, A. P., Gulley, M. R., & Cunningham, M. R. (1990). Support seeking in personal relationships. Special issue: Predicting, activating and facilitating social support. *Journal of Social and Personal Relationships, 7*(4), 531-540.

Barnard, K. E., Snyder, C., & Spietz, A. (1984). Supportive measures for high-risk infants. *Birth Defects: Original Article Series, 20*(5), 291-329.

Baron, R. A., & Byrne, D. (1977). *Social psychology: Understanding human interaction.* Boston: Allyn & Bacon.

Barrera, M. (1986). Distinctions between social support concepts, measures and models. *American Journal of Community Psychology, 14*(4), 435-447.

Barrera, M. (1991). Social support interventions and the third law of ecology. *American Journal of Community Psychology, 19*(1), 133-138.

Barrera, M., & Bacash, T. (1990). Recipient reactions to social support: Contributions of enacted support and network orientation. *Journal of Social and Personal Relationships, 7*(4), 541-551.

Barrera, M., Sandler, I., & Ramsay, T. (1981). Preliminary development of a scale of social support: Studies of college students. *American Journal of Community Psychology, 9*(4), 435-447.

Bass, D. M., Bowman, K., & Noelker, L. S. (1991). The influence of caregiving and bereavement support on adjusting to an older relative's death. *The Gerontologist, 31*(1), 32-42.

Baucom, D. H. (1987). Attribution in distressed relations: How can we explain them? In D. Perlman & S. Duck (Eds.), *Intimate relationships: Development, dynamics and deterioration* (pp. 177-206). Newbury Park, CA: Sage.

Baumgart, A. J. (1982). Nursing for a new century: A future framework. *Journal of Advanced Nursing, 7*, 19-23.

Beatty-Nelson, P. (1989). Social support, self-esteem, and depression in the institutionalized elderly. *Issues in Mental Health Nursing, 10*, 55-68.

Beck, A. *Depression: Clinical, perinatal and theorical aspects*. New York: Harper & Row.

Belle, D. (1987). Gender differences in the social moderators of stress. In R. C. Barnett, L. Biener, & G. Baruch (Eds.), *Gender and stress* (pp. 257-277). New York: Free Press.

Benner, P. (1984). *From novice to expert*. Menlo Park, CA: Addison-Wesley.

Benner, P. (1985). *Heideggerian phenomenology*. Paper presented at Third Annual Scientific Meeting of the Society for Research in Nursing Education, San Francisco, CA.

Berkman, L. F. (1985). The relationship of social networks and social support to morbidity and mortality. In S. Cohen & S. L. Syme (Eds.), *Social support and health* (pp. 241-262). Orlando, FL: Academic Press.

Berkman, L. F., & Breslow, L. (1990). Health practices and mortality risk. In L. F. Berkman & L. Breslow (Eds.), *Health and ways of living* (pp. 113-160). New York: Oxford University Press.

Berkman, L. S., & Syme, S. L. (1979). Social networks, host resistance, and mortality: A nine-year follow-up study of Alameda County residents. *American Journal of Epidemiology, 109*(2), 186-204.

Bernard, H., Johnson, E., Killworth, P., McCarthy, C., Shelley, G., & Robinson, S. (1990). Comparing four different methods for measuring personal social networks. *Social Networks, 12*, 179-215.

Bernstein, R. J. (1976). *The restructuring of social and political theory*. New York: Harcourt Brace Jovanovich.

Betz, C. L., Unger, O. A., Frager, B., Test, L., & Smith, C. (1990). A survey of self-help groups in California for parents of children with chronic conditions. *Pediatric Nursing, 16*(3), 293-296.

Biegel, R. C., & Naparstek, A. J. (1982). *Community support systems and mental health*. New York: Springer.

Billings, A. G., & Moos, R. H. (1981). The role of coping resources in attenuating the stress of life events. *Journal of Behavioral Medicine, 7*, 139-157.

Birkel, R. C., & Jones, C. J. (1989). A comparison of the caregiving networks of dependent elderly individuals who are lucid and those who are demented. *The Gerontologist, 29*(1), 114-119.

Birkel, R. C., & Repucci, N. (1983). Social networks, information seeking, and the utilization of services. *American Journal of Community Psychology, 11*(2), 185-205.

Bizek, K. S., & Oermann, A. (1990). Study of educational experiences, support, and job satisfaction among critical care nurse preceptors. *Heart and Lung: The Journal of Critical Care, 19*(5), 439-444.

Black, R. B., & Drachman, D. (1985). Hospital social workers and self-help groups. *Health and Social Work, 10*, 95-103.

Black, R. B., & Weiss, J. (1990). Genetic support groups and social workers as partners. *Health and Social Work, 15*(2), 91-99.

Blaney, N. T., Goodkin, K., Morgan, R., Feaster, D., Miller, C., Szapocznik, J., & Eisdorfer, C. (1991). A stress-moderator model of distress in early HIV-1 infection:

Concurrent analysis of life events, hardiness and social support. *Journal of Psychosomatic Research, 35*(2-3), 297-305.

Blau, P. M. (1964). *Exchange and power in social life.* New York: John Wiley.

Blazer, D. G. (1982). Social support and mortality in an elderly population. *American Journal of Epidemiology, 115*, 684-694.

Bledstein, B. J. (1976). *The culture of professionalism.* New York: Norton.

Bliwise, N. G., & Lieberman, M. (1984). From professional help to self-help: An evaluation of therapeutic groups for the elderly. In A. Gartner & F. Riessman (Eds.), *The self-help revolution* (pp. 217-232). New York: Human Sciences Press.

Bloom, J. R. (1990). The relationship of social support and health. *Social Science and Medicine, 39*(5), 635-637.

Blumer, H. (1969). *Symbolic interactionism: Perspective and method.* Englewood Cliffs, NJ: Prentice Hall.

Boettcher, M., & Schiller, W. (1990). The use of a multidisciplinary group meeting for families of critically ill trauma patients. *Intensive Care Nursing, 6*(3), 129-137.

Borkman, T. (1976). Experiential knowledge: A new concept for the analysis of self-help groups. *Social Service Review, 50*, 445-454.

Borkman, T. (1982). *A social experiential model in programs for alcoholism recovery.* Rockville, MD: U.S. Department of Health and Human Services.

Borkman, T. (1984). Mutual self-help groups: Strengthening the selectively unsupportive personal and community networks of their members. In A. Gartner & F. Reissman (Eds.), *The self-help revolution* (pp. 205-215). New York: Human Sciences Press.

Borkman, T. (1990). Self-help groups at the turning point: Emerging egalitarian alliances with the formal health care system? *American Journal of Community Psychology, 18*(2), 321-332.

Boyce, W. T., Kay, M., & Uitti, C. (1988). The taxonomy of social support: An ethnographic analysis among adolescent mothers. *Social Science and Medicine, 26*(11), 1079-1085.

Boyle, J. S. (1989). Constructs of health promotion and wellness in a Salvadoran population. *Public Health Nursing, 6*(3), 129-134.

Braden, C. J. (1990). A test of the self-help model: Learned responses to chronic illness experience. *Nursing Research, 39*(1), 42-47.

Branckaerts, J. (1983). The Belgian Huntington League: A case study in the collaboration between professional and lay people in a self-help group. In S. Hatch & I. Kickbusch (Eds.), *Self-help and health in Europe* (pp.94-100). Copenhagen, Denmark: World Health Organization.

Brandt, P. A. (1984a). Clinical assessment of the social support of families with handicapped children. *Issues in Comprehensive Pediatric Nursing, 7*, 187-201.

Brandt, P. A. (1984b). Stress buffering effects of social support on maternal discipline. *Nursing Research, 33*(4), 229-234.

Brandt, P. A., & Weinert, C. (1981). The PRQ: A social support measure. *Nursing Research, 30*(5), 277-280.

Bramwell, L., & Whall, A. L. (1986). Effect of role clarity and empathy on support role performance and anxiety. *Nursing Research, 35*, 282-287.

Brehm, S. S., & Brehm, J. W. (1981). *Psychological reactance: A theory of freedom and control.* New York: Academic Press.

Bremer-Schulte, M. (1983). Self-help and medical education. In S. Hatch & I. Kickbusch (Eds.), *Self-help and health in Europe: New approaches in health care* (pp. 77-89). Copenhagen: World Health Organization.

Brenner, G. F., Norwell, N. R., & Limacher, M. (1989). Supportive and problematic social interactions: A social network analysis. *American Journal of Community Psychology, 12*(6), 831-836.

Brickman, P., Kidder, L. H., Coates, D., Rabinowitz, V., Cohn, E., & Karuza, J. (1983). The dilemmas of helping: Making aid fair and effective. In J. D. Fisher, D. Nadler, & B. M. DePaulo (Eds.), *New directions in helping: Vol. 1. Recipient reactions to aid* (pp. 18-51). New York: Academic Press.

Brickman, P., Rabinowitz, V., Karuza, J., Coates, D., Cohen, E., & Kidder, L. (1982). Models of helping and coping. *American Psychologist, 37*, 368-384.

Brink, P. J. (1987). Personal communication regarding an earlier version of a paper.

Brink, P. J., & Wood, M. J. (1983). *Basic steps in planning nursing research: From question to proposal.* Monterey, CA: Wadsworth.

Broadhead, W. E., Kaplan, B. H., James, S., Wagner, E., Schoenbach, V., Grimson, R., Heyden, S., Tibblin, G., & Gehlbach, S. (1983). The epidemiological evidence for a relationship between social support and health. *American Journal of Epidemiology, 117*, 521-536.

Brock, A. M.., & O'Sullivan, P. (1985). A study to determine what variables predict institutionalization of elderly people. *Journal of Advanced Nursing, 10*, 533-537.

Brown, B. B. (1978). Social and psychological correlates of help-seeking behavior among urban adults. *American Journal of Community Psychology, 6*, 425-439.

Brown, G. W., & Bifulco, A. (1985). Social support, life events and depression. In I. G. Sarason & B. R. Sarason (Eds.), *Social support: Theory, research, application* (pp. 349-370). Dordrecht, The Netherlands: Martinus Nijhoff.

Brown, L. D., & Tandon, R. (1983). Ideology and political economy in inquiry: Action research and participatory research. *The Journal of Applied Behavioral Science, 19*(3), 277-294.

Brown, M. A. (1986a). Social support during pregnancy: A unidimensional or multidimensional construct? *Nursing Research, 35*(1), 4-9.

Brown, M. A. (1986b). Social support, stress and health: A comparison of expectant mothers and fathers. *Nursing Research, 35*, 72-76.

Brownell, A., & Shumaker, S. A. (1984). Social support: An introduction to a complex phenomenon. *Journal of Social Issues, 40*(4), 1-9.

Brownell, A., & Shumaker, S. A. (1985). Where do we go from here? The policy implications of social support. *Journal of Social Issues, 41*(1), 111-121.

Browner, C. H. (1987). Job stress and health: The role of social support at work. *Research in Nursing and Health, 10*, 93-100.

Bruera, E., Kuehn, N., Emery, B., MacMillan, K., & Hanson, J. (1990). Social and demographic characteristics of patients admitted to a palliative care unit. *Journal of Palliative Care, 6*(4), 16-20.

Bryant, B. K. (1985). The neighbourhood walk: Sources of support in middle childhood. *Monographs in Sociology Research and Child Development, 50*, 210.

Burgess, A. W., & Holmstrom, L. L. (1978). Recovery from rape and prior life stress. *Research in Nursing and Health, 1*, 165-174.

Burleson, B. R. (1982). The development of comforting communication skills in childhood and adolescence. *Child Development, 53*, 1578-1588.

Canadian Nurses Association. (1988). *Health for all Canadians: A call for health care reform.* Ottawa, Ontario, Canada: Author.

Cantor, M. H. (1979). Neighbours and friends: An overlooked resource in the informal support system. *Research on Aging, 1,* 434-463.

Caplan, G. (1974). *Support systems and community mental health.* New York: Behavioral Publications.

Caplan, G. (1976). *Support systems and mutual help: Multidisciplinary exploration.* New York: Grune & Stratton.

Caplan, G. (1981). Mastery of stress in psychosocial aspects. *American Journal of Psychiatry, 138,* 413-420.

Capuzzi, C. (1989). Maternal attachment to handicapped infants and the relationship to social support. *Research in Nursing and Health, 12,* 161-167.

Cassel, J. (1974). Psychosocial processes and stress: Theoretical formulation. *International Journal of Health Services, 4*(3), 471-482.

Cassel, J. (1976). The contribution of the social environment to host resistance. *American Journal of Epidemiology, 104*(2), 107-123.

Cawley, M., Kostic, J., & Cappello, A. (1990). Informational and psychosocial needs of women choosing conservative surgery/primary radiation for early stage breast cancer. *Cancer Nursing, 13*(2), 90-94.

Chapman, N. J., & Pancoast, D. L. (1985). Working with the informal helping networks of the elderly: The experiences of three programs. *Journal of Social Issues, 41*(1), 47-63.

Charlesworth, M. (1982). *Science, non-science and pseudo-science.* Geelong, Victoria, Australia: Deakin University Press.

Cherniss, C., & Cherniss, D. S. (1987). Professional involvement in self-help groups for parents of high-risk newborns. *American Journal of Community Psychology, 15*(4), 435-444.

Chesler, M. A. (1991). Participatory action research with self-help groups: An alternative paradigm for inquiry and action. *American Journal of Community Psychology, 19*(5), 757-768.

Chesler, M. A., & Barbarin, D. A. (1984). Difficulties of providing help in a crisis: Relationships between parents of children with cancer and their friends. *Journal of Social Issues, 40*(4), 113-134.

Chesler, M. A., & Yoak, M. (1984). Self-help groups for parents of children with cancer. In H. B. Roback (Ed.), *Helping patients and their families cope with medical problems* (pp. 481-526). San Francisco: Jossey-Bass.

Chinn, P. (1983). Nursing theory development: Where we have been and where we are going. In N. L. Chaska (Ed.), *The nursing profession: A time to speak* (pp. 394-405). New York: McGraw-Hill.

Chinn, P., & Jacobs, L. (1987). *Theory and nursing: A systematic approach.* St. Louis, MO: C. V. Mosby.

Chiriboga, D. A., Jenkins, G., & Bailey, J. (1983). Stress and coping among hospice nurses: Test of an analytic model. *Nursing Research, 32*(5), 294-299.

Chopoorian, T. J. (1986). Reconceptualizing the environment. In P. Moccia (Ed.), *New approaches to theory development* (pp. 39-54). New York: National League for Nursing.

Christopherson-Yates, B. (1989). Stress and social support during recovery from a cardiac illness event. *The Oklahoma Nurse, 1,* 7.

Clark, M. S. (1983). Reactions to aid in communal and exchange relationships. In J. D. Fisher, D. Nadler, & B. M. DePaulo (Eds.), *New directions in helping: Vol. 1. Recipient reactions to aid* (pp. 281-305). New York: Academic Press.

Clark, M. S. (1984). A distinction between two types of relationships and its implications for development. In J. C. Masters & K. Yarkin-Levin (Eds.), *Boundary areas in social and developmental psychology* (pp. 241-270). New York: Academic Press.

Clark, M. S., & Reis, H. T. (1988). Interpersonal processes in close relationships. In M. R. Rosenzweig & L. W. Porter (Eds.), *Annual Review of Psychology, 39*, 609-672.

Clarke, M. (1986). Action and reflection: Practice and theory in nursing. *Journal of Advanced Nursing, 11*, 3-11.

Clements, D. B., Copeland, L. G., & Loftus, M. (1990). Critical times for families with a chronically ill child. *Pediatric Nursing, 16*(2), 157-162.

Coates, D., & Winston, J. (1985). Counteracting the deviance of depression: Peer support groups for victims. *Journal of Social Issues, 39*(1), 169-194.

Cobb, S. (1976). Social support as a moderator of life stress. *Psychosomatic Medicine, 38*, 300-314.

Cochran, M. M., & Brassard, J. A. (1979). Child development and personal networks. *Child Development, 50*, 601-616.

Cohen, J. H. (1990). Community nurse executives' psychologic well-being: Relationships among stressors, social support, coping and optimism. *Public Health Nursing, 7*(4), 194-203.

Cohen, J. L. (1985). Strategy or identity: New theoretical paradigms and contemporary social movements. *Social Research, 52*(4), 663-716.

Cohen, R. Y. (1988). Mobilizing support for weight loss through work-site competitions. In B. H. Gottlieb (Ed.), *Marshalling social support: Formats, processes, and effects* (pp. 241-264). Newbury Park, CA: Sage.

Cohen, S., & McKay, G. (1984). Social support, stress and the buffering hypothesis: A theoretical analysis. In A. Baum, J. E. Singer, & S. E. Taylor (Eds.), *Handbook of psychology and health* (Vol. 4). Hillsdale, NJ: Lawrence Erlbaum.

Cohen, S., Mermelstein, R., Kamarck, T., & Hoberman, H. M. (1985). Measuring the functional components of social support. In I. Sarason & B. Sarason (Eds.), *Social support: Theory, research and applications* (pp. 73-94). Dordrecht, The Netherlands: Martinus Nijhoff.

Cohen, S., & Syme, S. L. (1985). Issues in the study and application of social support. In S. Cohen & S. L. Syme (Eds.), *Social support and health* (pp. 3-22). Orlando, FL: Academic Press.

Cohen, S., & Wills, T. A. (1985). Stress, social support and the buffering hypothesis. *Psychological Bulletin, 98*(2), 310-357.

Cohen-Mansfield, J. (1989). Sources of satisfaction and stress in nursing home caregivers: Preliminary results. *Journal of Advanced Nursing, 14*, 383-388.

Collins, C., Given, B., & Berry, D. (1989). Longitudinal studies as intervention. *Nursing Research, 38*(4), 251-253.

Comi-McCloskey, K. (1990). Two requirements for job contentment: Autonomy and social integration. *Image: Journal of Nursing Scholarship, 22*(3), 140-143.

Compas, B. (1987). Coping with stress during childhood and adolescence. *Psychological Bulletin, 101*(8), 393-403.

Conway, M. E. (1986). Toward greater specificity in defining nursing's metaparadigm. *Advances in Nursing Science, 9*, 73-81.

Cook, L. (1990). Nurses in crisis: A support group based on Travelbee's Nursing Theory. *Nursing and Health Care, 10*(4), 203-205.

Cox, C. (1986). The interaction model of client health behavior: Application to the study of community-based elders. *Advances in Nursing Science, 9*(1), 40-57.

Coyne, J. C., & Bulger, N. (1990). Doing without support as an explanatory concept. *Journal of Social and Clinical Psychology, 9*(1), 148-158.

Coyne, J. C., & DeLongis, A. (1986). Going beyond social support: The role of social relationships in adaptation. *Journal of Consulting and Clinical Psychology, 54*, 454-460.

Coyne, J. C., & Downey, G. (1991). Social factors and psychopathology: Stress, social support, and coping processes. *Annual Review of Psychology, 42*, 401-425.

Coyne, J. C., Ellard, J. H., & Smith, D. A. F. (1990). Social support, interdependence, and the dilemmas of helping. In B. R. Sarason, I. G. Sarason, & G. R. Pierce (Eds.), *Social support: An interactional view* (pp. 129-149). New York: John Wiley.

Coyne, J. C., Wortman, C. B., & Lehman, D. R. (1988). The other side of support: Emotional overinvolvement and miscarried helping. In B. H. Gottlieb (Ed.), *Marshalling social support: Formats, processes, and effects* (pp. 305-330). Newbury Park, CA: Sage.

Cranley, M. S. (1984). Social support as a factor in the development of parents' attachment to their unborn. *Birth Defects: Original Article Series, 20*,(5) 99-124.

Cronenwett, L. R. (1980). Elements and outcomes of a postpartum support group program. *Research in Nursing and Health, 3*, 33-41.

Cronenwett, L. R. (1983). When and how people help: Theoretical issues and evidence. In P. L. Chinn (Ed.), *Advances in nursing theory development* (pp. 251-270). Rockville, MD: Aspen.

Cronenwett, L. R. (1984). Social networks and social support of primigravada mothers and fathers. *Birth Defects: Original Article Series, 20*(5), 167-203.

Cronenwett, L. R. (1985a). Network structure, social support and psychological outcomes of pregnancy. *Nursing Research, 34*(2), 93-99.

Cronenwett, L. R. (1985b). Parental network structure and perceived support after birth of first child. *Nursing Research, 34*(6), 347-352.

Cronenwett, L. R., & Brickman, P. (1983). Models of helping and coping in childbirth. *Nursing Research, 32*(3), 84-88.

Cronenwett, L. R., & Kunst-Wilson, W. (1981). Stress, social support and the transition to fatherhood. *Nursing Research, 30*(4), 196-201.

Cronin-Stubbs, D., & Brophy, E. (1985). Burnout: Can social support save the psych nurse? *Journal of Psychosocial Nursing, 23*(7), 9-13.

Cronin-Stubbs, D., & Rooks, C. A. (1985). The stress, social support, and burnout of critical care nurses: The results of research. *Heart and Lung: The Journal of Critical Care, 14*(1), 31-39.

Cunningham, A. J. (1981). Mind, body and immune response. In R. Ader (Ed.), *Psychoneuroimmunology* (pp. 609-617). New York: Academic Press.

Cutrona, C. E. (1990). Stress and social support: In search of optimal matching. *Journal of Social and Clinical Psychology, 9*(1), 3-14.

Cutrona, C., Russell, D., & Rose, J. (1986). Social support and adaptation to stress by the elderly. *Journal of Psychological Aging, 1*, 47-54.

D'Augelli, A. R., & Ehrlick, R. P. (1982). Evaluation of a community-based system for training natural helpers: II. Effects on informal helping activities. *American Journal of Community Psychology, 10*(4), 447-456.

Dahlem, N. W., Zimet, G. D., & Walker, R. R. (1991). The multidimensional scale of perceived support: A confirmation study. *Journal of Clinical Psychology, 47*(6), 756-761.

Dakof, G. A., & Taylor, S. E. (1990). Victims' perceptions of social support: What is helpful from whom? *Journal of Personality and Social Psychology, 58*(1), 80-89.

Dallmayr, F. R., & McCarthy, T. A. (1977). *Understanding and social inquiry.* Notre Dame, IN: University of Notre Dame Press.

Darko, D. F. (1986). A brief tour of psychoneuroimmunology. *Annual Allergy, 57,* 233-238.

Davies, B., & Oberle, K. (1990). Dimensions of the supportive role of the nurse in palliative care. *Oncology Nursing Forum, 17*(1), 87-94.

Dean, P. G. (1989). Expanding our sights to include social networks. *Nursing and Health Care, 12,* 545-550.

DePaulo, B. M. (1982). Social-psychological processes in informal help seeking. In T. A. Wills (Ed.), *Basic processes in helping relationships* (pp. 255-280). New York: Academic Press.

Derber, C. (1982). *Professionals as workers: Mental labor in advanced capitalism.* Boston: G. K. Hall.

Diekmann, J. (1988). An evaluation of selected I Can Cope programs by registered participants. *Cancer Nursing, 11*(5), 274-282.

Dignam, A., & West, S. (1988). Social support in the workplace: Tests of six theoretical models. *American Journal of Community Psychology, 16*(5), 701-724.

Dimond, M. (1979). Social support and adaptation to chronic illness: The case of maintenance dialysis. *Research in Nursing and Health, 2,* 101-108.

Dimond, M. (1985). A review and critique of the concepts of social support. In R. A. O'Brien (Ed.), *Social support and health: New directions for theory and research* (pp. 1-32). Rochester, NY: University of Rochester Press.

Dimond, M., & Jones, S. (1983). Social support: A review and theoretical integration. In P. Chinn (Ed.), *Advances in nursing theory development* (pp. 235-249). Rockville, MD: Aspen.

Dingwall, R., & Lewis, P. (1983). *The sociology of the professions.* New York: St. Martin's.

Dixon, J. K. (1981). Group self identification and physical handicap: Implications for patient support groups. *Research in Nursing and Health, 4,* 299-308.

Donaldson, S. K., & Crowley, D. M. (1978). The discipline of nursing. *Nursing Outlook, 26,* 113-120.

Donati, P. R. (1984). Organization between movement and instruction. *Social Science Information, 23*(4), 837-859.

Dooley, D. (1985). Causal inference in the study of social support. In S. Cohen & S. Syme (Eds.), *Social support and health* (pp. 109-125). Orlando, FL: Academic Press.

Dormire, S. L., Strauss, S. S., & Clarke, B. A. (1989). Social support and adaptation to the parent role in first-time adolescent mothers. *Journal of Obstetric, Gynecologic, and Neonatal Nursing, 18*(4), 327-336.

Downs, F. (1989). Glue [Editorial]. *Nursing Research, 38*(3), 133.

Doyle, E., & Straub, V. W. (1985). An intervention to improve social supports in high risk populations. In R. A. O'Brien (Ed.), *Social support and health: New directions for theory development and research* (pp. 221-224). Rochester, NY: University of Rochester Press.

Dracup, K. (1985). A controlled trial of couples' group counseling in cardiac rehabilitation. *Journal of Cardiopulmonary Rehabilitation, 5,* 436-442.

Duffy, M. E. (1989). The primary support received by recently divorced mothers. *Western Journal of Nursing Research, 11*(6), 676-693.

Dulaney, P., Crawford, V., & Turner, G. (1990). A comprehensive education and support program for women experiencing hysterectomies. *Journal of Obstetric, Gynecologic, and Neonatal Nursing, 19*(4), 319-325.

Duldt, B., & Giffin, K. (1985). *Theoretical perspectives for nursing.* Boston: Little, Brown.

Dunkel-Schetter, C., & Bennett, T. (1990). Differentiating the cognitive and behavioral aspects of social support. In B. R. Sarason, I. B. Sarason, & G. R. Pierce (Eds.), *Social support: An interactional view* (pp. 208, 267-296). New York: John Wiley.

Dunkel-Schetter, C., Folkman, S., & Lazarus, R. S. (1987). Correlates of social support receipt. *Journal of Personality and Social Psychology, 53,* 71-80.

Dunkel-Schetter, C., & Skokan, L. (1990). Determinants of social support provision in personal relationships. *Journal of Social and Personal Relationships, 7*(4), 437-450.

Dunkel-Schetter, C., & Wortman, C. B. (1985). The role of social support in adaptation and recovery from physical illness. In S. Cohen & S. L. Syme (Eds.), *Social support and health* (pp. 281-302). Orlando, FL: Academic Press.

Durlak, J. (1979). Comparative effectiveness of paraprofessional and professional helpers. *Psychology Bulletin, 86,* 80-92.

Eckberg, D. L., & Hill, L. (1979). The paradigm concept and sociology: A critical review. *American Sociological Review, 44,* 925-937.

Eckenrode, J. (1983). The mobilization of social supports: Some individual constraints. *American Journal of Community Psychology, 11*(5), 509-528.

Eckenrode, J., & Gore, S. (1981). Stressful events and social supports: The significance of context. In B. H. Gottlieb (Ed.), *Social networks and social supports* (pp. 43-68). Beverly Hills, CA: Sage.

Eckenrode, J., & Gore, S. (1990). *Stress between work and family* (pp. 55-59). New York: Plenum.

Ede, K. (1985). The new social movements: Moral crusaders, political pressure groups or social movements? *Social Research, 52*(4), 869-890.

Elliott, S. A., Sanjack, M., & Leverton, T. J. (1988). Parents' groups in pregnancy: A preventive intervention for postnatal depression? In B. H. Gottlieb (Ed.), *Marshalling social support: Formats, processes, and effects* (pp. 87-110). Newbury Park, CA: Sage.

Ellis, R. (1982). Conceptual issues in nursing. *Nursing Outlook, 30,* 406-410.

Emerick, R. E. (1991). The politics of psychiatric self-help: Political factions, interactional support and group longevity in a social movement. *Social Science and Medicine, 32*(10), 1121-1128.

Epp, J. (1986). *Achieving health for all: A framework for health promotion.* Ottawa, Ontario: Health and Welfare Canada.

Farquharson, A. (1987). *Professional involvement with self-help groups: Experiential knowledge and the member role or a tale of two icebergs.* Paper presented at the National Meeting on Self-Help/Mutual Aid, Ottawa, Ontario, Canada.

Farquharson, A., & Cardinal, J. (1989). *A guide to the competency profile: Human service professionals working with self-help mutual aid groups.* Unpublished manuscript. University of Victoria, British Columbia, Canada.

Fawcett, J. (1989). *Analysis and evaluation of conceptual models of nursing.* (2nd ed.) Philadelphia: F. A. Davis.

Feinberg, W. (1983). *Understanding education: Toward a reconstruction of educational inquiry*. Cambridge, UK: Cambridge University Press.

Ferketich, S. L., & Mercer, R. T. (1990). Effects of antepartal stress on health status during early motherhood. *Scholarly Inquiry for Nursing Practice: An International Journal, 4*(2), 127-149.

Festinger, L. (1954). A theory of social comparison. *Human Relations, 1*, 117-140.

Field, P., & Morse, J. (1985). *Nursing research: The application of qualitative approaches*. Rockville, MD: Aspen.

Field, P., & Renfrew, M. (1991). Teaching and support: Nursing input in the postpartum period. *International Journal of Nursing Studies, 28*(2), 131-144.

Firth, H., McIntee, J., McKeown, P., & Britton, P. (1986). Interpersonal support amongst nurses at work. *Journal of Advanced Nursing, 11*, 273-282.

Fisher, J. D., Goff, B. A., Nadler, A., & Chinsky, J. M. (1988). Social psychological influences on help seeking and support from peers. In B. H. Gottlieb (Ed.), *Marshalling social support: Formats, processes, and effects* (pp. 267-304). Newbury Park, CA: Sage.

Fisher, J. D., & Nadler, A. (1982). Determinants of recipient reaction to aid: Donor recipient similarity and perceived dimensions of problems. In T. A. Wills (Ed.), *Basic processes in helping relationships* (pp. 131-154). New York: Academic Press.

Fisher, J. D., Nadler, A., & Whitcher-Alagna, S. (1983). Four theoretical approaches for conceptualizing reactions to aid. In J. D. Fisher, D. Nadler, & B. M. DePaulo (Eds.), *New directions in helping: Vol. 1. Recipient reactions to aid* (pp. 52-85). New York: Academic Press.

Flaherty, J., & Richman, J. (1989). Gender differences in the perception and utilization of social support: Theoretical perspectives and an empirical test. *Social Science and Medicine, 28*(12), 1221-1228.

Flaskerud, J. H., & Halloran, E. J. (1980). Areas of agreement in nursing theory development. *Advances in Nursing Science, 2*(1), 1-7.

Florian, V., & Krulik, T. (1991). Loneliness and social support of mothers of chronically ill children. *Social Science and Medicine, 32*(11), 1291-1296.

Folkman, S., & Lazarus, R. S. (1980). An analysis of coping in a middle-aged community sample. *Journal of Health and Social Behavior, 21*(9), 219-239.

Fong, C. M. (1990). Role overload, social support and burnout among nurse educators. *Journal of Nursing Education, 29*(3), 102-108.

Foote, A. W., Piazza, D., & Holcombe, J. (1990). Hope, self-esteem and social support in persons with multiple sclerosis. *Journal of Neuroscience Nursing, 22*(3), 155-159.

Ford, G., & Procidano, M. (1990). The relationship of self actualization to social support, life stress and adjustment. *Social Behavior and Personality, 18*(1), 41-51.

Fox, B. H. (1981). Psychosocial factors and the immune system in human cancer. In R. Ader (Ed.), *Psychoneuroimmunology* (pp. 103-157). New York: Academic Press.

Frey, M. (1989). Social support and health: A theoretical formulation derived from King's Conceptual Framework. *Nursing Science Quarterly, 2*(3), 138-148.

Fridlund, B., Liddell, E., & Larsson, P. (1989). A caring perspective on rehabilitation after myocardial infarction. *Scandinavian Journal of Caring Science, 3*(3), 129-135.

Friedman, M. M. (1985). The impact of stress and social support on family conflict among Anglo and Latino families with childhood cancer. In R. A. O'Brien (Ed.), *Social support and health: New directions for theory and research* (pp. 23-31). Rochester, NY: University of Rochester Press.

Friedson, E. (1983). The theory of professions: State of the art. In R. Dingwall & P. Lewis (Eds.), *The sociology of the professions* (pp. 19-37). New York: St. Martin's.

Froland, C. (1980). Formal and informal care: Discontinuities in a continuum. *Social Services Review, 50,* 572-587.

Froland, C., Pancoast, D., Chapman, N., & Kimboko, P. (1981). *Helping networks and human services.* Beverly Hills, CA: Sage.

Fruehwirth, E. S. (1989). An application of Johnson's behavioral model: A case study. *Journal of Community Health Nursing, 6*(2), 61-71.

Fuller, S., & Larson, S. (1980). Life events, emotional support, and health of older people. *Research in Nursing and Health, 3,* 81-89.

Gambosi, J., & Ulreich, S. (1990). Recovering from cancer: A nursing intervention program recognizing survivorship. *Oncology Nursing Forum, 17*(2), 215-219.

Garbarino, J. (1980). *Protecting children from abuse and neglect: Developing and maintaining effective support systems for families.* San Francisco: Jossey-Bass.

Gardner, K. G., & Wheeler, E. C. (1987). Patients' perceptions of support. *Western Journal of Nursing Research, 9,* 115-131.

Gartner, A., & Riessman, F. (1984). *The self-help revolution.* New York: Human Sciences.

Garvin, B. J., & Kennedy, C. W. (1990). Interpersonal communication between nurses and patients. *Annual Review of Nursing Research, 8,* 213-234.

Geary, P. A. (1989). Stress and social support in the experience of monitoring apneic infants. *Clinical Nurse Specialist, 3*(3), 119-125.

Gierszeweski, S. A. (1983). The relationship of weight loss, locus of control and social support. *Nursing Research, 32,* 43-47.

Glaser, R., Kiecolt-Glaser, J. K., Speicher, C. E., & Holliday, J. E. (1985). Stress, loneliness, and changes in herpes virus latency. *Journal of Behavioral Medicine, 8,* 249-260.

Glennon, T., & Smith, B. (1990). Questions asked by patients and their support groups during family conferences on patient rehabilitation units. *Archives of Physical and Medical Rehabilitation, 71*(9), 699-702.

Goetzel, R. Z., Shelov, S., & Croen, L. G. (1983). Evaluating medical student self-help support groups: A general systems model. *Small Group Behavior, 14*(3), 337-352.

Goldklang, D. S. (1991). Research workshop on methodological issues in evaluating preventive interventions using mutual support. *American Journal of Community Psychology, 19*(5), 789-795.

Goldsmith, D., & Parks, M. (1990). Communication strategies for managing the risks of seeking social support. In S. Duck (Ed.), *Personal relationships and social support* (pp. 104-121). London: Sage.

Gonzalez, J. T. (1990). Factors relating to frequency of breast self-examination among low-income Mexican American women. *Cancer Nursing, 13*(3), 134-142.

Gonzalez, U., Goepperinger, J., & Lorig, V. (1990). Four psychological theories and their application to patient education and clinical practice. *Arthritis Care and Research, 3*(3), 132-143.

Gore, S. (1985). Social support and styles of coping with stress. In S. Cohen & S. L. Syme (Eds.), *Social support and health* (pp. 263-278). Orlando, FL: Academic Press.

Gottlieb, B. H. (1981). Preventive interventions involving social networks and social support. In B. H. Gottlieb (Ed.), *Social networks and social support* (pp. 201-232). Beverly Hills, CA: Sage.

Gottlieb, B. H. (1982a). Mutual help groups: Members' views of their benefits and of roles for professionals. *Prevention in Human Services, 1,* 55-67.

Gottlieb, B. H. (1982b). Social support in the workplace. In D. E. Biegel & A. J. Naparstek, *Community support systems and mental health: Practice, policy, and research* (pp. 37-53). New York: Springer.

Gottlieb, B. H. (1983). *Social support strategies: Guidelines for mental health practice*. Beverly Hills, CA: Sage.

Gottlieb, B. H. (1985a). Marshaling and augmenting social support for medical patients and their families. In R. A. O'Brien (Ed.), *Social support and health: New directions for theory and research* (pp. 107-148). Rochester, NY: University of Rochester Press.

Gottlieb, B. H. (1985b). Social networks and social support: An overview of research, practice and policy implications. *Health Education Quarterly, 12*(1), 5-22.

Gottlieb, B. H. (1985c). Theory into practice: Issues that surface in planning interventions which mobilize support. In I. G. Sarason & B. R. Sarason (Eds.), *Social support: Theory, research, application* (pp. 417-438). Dordrecht, The Netherlands: Martinus Nijhoff.

Gottlieb, B. H. (1987). Using social support to promote mental health. *Journal of Primary Prevention, 8*, 49-70.

Gottlieb, B. H. (1988a). Marshaling social support: The state of the art in research and practice. In B. H. Gottlieb (Ed.), *Marshaling social support: Formats, processes, and effects* (pp. 11-52). Newbury Park, CA: Sage.

Gottlieb, B. H. (1988b). Support interventions: A typology and agenda for research. In S. Duck (Ed.), *Handbook of personal relationships* (pp. 519-541). Chichester, UK: John Wiley.

Gottlieb, B. H. (1989). A contextual perspective on stress in family care of the elderly. *Canadian Psychology, 30*(3), 596-607.

Gottlieb, B. H. (1991). Peer telephone dyads: Putting conclusions on hold. *American Journal of Community Psychology, 19*(1), 123-132.

Gottlieb, B. H., & Farquharson, A. (1985). Blueprint for a curriculum on social support. *Social Policy, 15*(3), 31-34.

Gottlieb, B. H., & Selby, P. M. (1989). Social support and mental health: A review of the literature. National Health Research Development Program (NHRDP) unpublished funded review. University of Guelph, Guelph, Ontario, Canada.

Gottlieb, B. H., & Wagner, F. (1991). Stress and support processes in close relationships. In J. Eckenrode (Ed.), *The social context of coping* (pp. 165-188). New York: Plenum.

Gottschalk, L. A. (1983). Vulnerability to stress. *American Journal of Psychotherapy, 1*, 5-23.

Gouldner, A. W. (1960). The norm of reciprocity: A preliminary statement. *American Sociological Review, 25*, 161-178.

Gourash, N. (1978). Help-seeking: A review of the literature. *American Journal of Community Psychology, 6*(5), 413-423.

Greenberg, M. S., & Westcott, D. R. (1983). Indebtedness as a mediator of reactions to aid. In J. D. Fisher, D. Nadler, & B. M. DePaulo (Eds.), *New directions in helping: Vol. 1. Recipient reactions to aid* (pp. 86-133). New York: Academic Press.

Griffith, J. (1985). Social support providers: Who are they? Where are they met? and the relationship of network characteristics to psychological distress. *Basic and Applied Social Psychology, 6*(1), 41-60.

Gundelach, P. (1984). Social transformations and new forms of voluntary associations. *Social Science Information, 23*(6), 1049-1081.

Haberman-Cohen, J. (1990). Community nurses executives' psychologic well-being: Relationships among stressors, social support, coping, and optimism. *Public Health Nursing, 7*(4), 194-203.

Hall, A., & Wellman, B. (1985). Social networks and social support. In S. Cohen & S. L. Syme (Eds.), *Social support and health* (pp. 23-41). Orlando, FL: Academic Press.

Hall, L. A., Schaefer, E. S., & Greenberg, R. S. (1987). Quality and quantity of social support as correlates of psychosomatic symptoms in mothers with young children. *Research in Nursing and Health, 10,* 39-47.

Halm, M. (1990). Effects of support groups on anxiety of family members during critical times. *Families in Critical Care, 19*(1), 62-71.

Hammer, M. (1983). Core and extended social networks in relation to health and illness. *Social Science and Medicine, 17,* 405-411.

Hanson, C. L., Herggeler, S. W., & Burghen, G. A. (1987). Social competence and parental support as mediators of the link between stress and metabolic control in adolescents with insulin-dependent diabetes mellitus. *Journal of Consulting and Clinical Psychology, 55,* 529-533.

Hanucharurnkul, S. (1989). Predictors of self-care in cancer patients receiving radiotherapy. *Cancer Nursing, 12*(1), 21-27.

Hardy, M. E. (1986). Identifying the place of theoretical frameworks in an evolving discipline. *Journal of Advanced Nursing, 11,* 103-107.

Harris, H. (1989). Reviewing nursing stress according to a proposed coping-adaptation framework. *Advances in Nursing Science, 11*(2), 12-28.

Hart, G., Mann, K., & Stewart, M. (1991). *The support needs of persons with hemophilia and AIDS or HIV related illness and of their family caregivers.* Unpublished report to National Health Research Development Program, Ottawa, Ontario, Canada.

Hatch, S., & Kickbusch, I. (1983). *Self-help and health in Europe.* Copenhagen: World Health Organization.

Hatfield, E., & Sprecher, S. (1983). Equity theory and recipient reactions to aid. In J. D. Fisher, D. Nadler, & B. M. Depaulo (Eds.), *New directions in helping: Vol. 1. Recipient reactions to aid* (pp. 113-143). New York: Academic Press.

Heider, F. (1958). *The psychology of interpersonal relations.* New York: John Wiley.

Heiney, S., Ruffin, J., Ettinger, R. S., & Ettinger, S. (1988). The effects of group therapy on adolescents with cancer. *Journal of the Association of Oncology Nurses, 5*(3), 20-24.

Heiney, S., & Wells, L. (1989). Strategies for organizing and maintaining successful support groups. *Oncology Nursing Forum, 16*(6), 803-809.

Heller, K. (1990). Social and community intervention. *Annual Review of Psychology, 41,* 141-168.

Heller, K., & Mansbach, W. E. (1984). The multifaceted nature of social support in a community sample of elderly women. *Journal of Social Issues, 40*(4), 99-112.

Heller, K., Price, R. H., & Hogg, J. R. (1990). The role of social support in community and clinical interventions. In B. R. Sarason, I. B. Sarason, & G. R. Pierce (Eds.), *Social support: An interactional view* (pp. 481-508). New York: John Wiley.

Heller, K., & Swindle, R. (1983). Social networks, perceived social support, and coping with stress. In R. Felner, L. Jason, J. Moritsugu, & S. Farber (Eds.), *Preventive psychology* (pp. 87-103). New York: Pergamon.

Heller, K., Swindle, R., & Dusenbury, L. (1986). Component social support processes: Comments and integration. *Journal of Consulting and Clinical Psychology, 54*(4), 466-470.

Heller, K., Thompson, M., Trueba, P., Hogg, J., & Vlachos-Weber, I. (1991). Peer support telephone dyads for elderly women: Was this the wrong intervention? *American Journal of Community Psychology, 19*(1), 53-74.

Heller, K., Thompson, M., Vlachos-Weber, I., Steffen, A., & Trueba, P. (1991). Support interventions for older adults: Confidante relationships, perceived family support, and meaningful role activity. *American Journal of Community Psychology, 19*(1), 139-143.

Henderson, A. D. (1989). Use of social support in a transition house for abused women. *Health Care for Women International, 10*, 61-73.

Hermalin, J., Melendez, L., Kamarch, T., Klevens, F., Ballen, E., & Gordon, M. (1979). Enhancing primary prevention: The marriage of self-help groups and formal health care delivery systems. *Journal of Clinical Child Psychology, 8*(2), 125-129.

Hermansen-Williams, M. (1990). The self-help movement in head injury. *Rehabilitation Nursing, 15*(6), 311-315.

Hersey, J. C., Klibanoff, L. S., Lam, D., & Taylor, R. (1984). Promoting social support: The impact of California "friends can be good medicine campaign." *Health Education Quarterly, 11*(3), 293-311.

Hewat, R. J., & Ellis, D. J. (1984). Breastfeeding as a maternal-child team effort: Women's perceptions. *Health Care for Women International, 5*, 437-452.

Higgins, P. G., & Dicharry, E. K. (1991). Measurement issues addressing social support with Navajo women. *Western Journal of Nursing Research, 13*(2), 242-255.

Hilbert, G. A. (1985). Spouse support and myocardial infarction patient compliance. *Nursing Research, 34*, 217-220.

Hilbert, G. A., & Allen, L. R. (1985). The effect of social support on educational outcomes. *Journal of Nursing Education, 24*(2), 48-52.

Hinds, C. (1985). The needs of families who care for patients with cancer at home. Are we meeting them? *Journal of Advanced Nursing, 10*, 575-581.

Hirose, T., & Ueda, R. (1990). Long-term follow-up study of cerebral palsy children and coping behavior of parents. *Journal of Advanced Nursing, 15*, 762-770.

Hirsch, B., & David, T. (1983). Social networks and work/nonwork life: Action research with nurse managers. *American Journal of Community Psychology, 11*(5), 493-507.

Hobfoll, S. E., & Freedy, J. R. (1990). The availability and effective use of social support. *Journal of Social and Clinical Psychology, 9*(1), 91-103.

Hobfoll, S. E., & Stokes, J. P. (1988). The process and mechanics of social support. In S. Duck, D. F. Hay, S. E. Hobfoll, W. Ickes, & B. M. Montgomery (Eds.), *Handbook of personal relationships: Theory, research and interventions* (pp. 497-517). London: John Wiley.

Hodnett, E. D., & Osborn, R. W. (1989a). Effects of continuous intrapartum professional support on childbirth outcomes. *Research in Nursing and Health, 12*, 289-297.

Hodnett, E. D., & Osborn, R. W. (1989b). A randomized trial of the effects of monitrice support during labor: Mothers' views two to four weeks postpartum. *Birth, 16*(4), 177-183.

Hoff, L. E. (1985). The influence of social network factors during and after battering. In R. A. O'Brien (Ed.), *Social support and health: New directions for theory and research* (pp. 185-189). Rochester, NY: University of Rochester Press.

Holaday, B. (1987). Patterns of interaction between mothers and their chronically ill infants. *Maternal-Child Nursing Journal, 16*, 29-45.

Holahan, C. J., & Moos, R. H. (1982). Social support and adjustment: Predictive benefits of social climate indices. *American Journal of Community Psychology, 10*(4), 403-413.
Homans, G. C. (1961). *Social behavior: Its elementary forms.* New York: Harcourt, Brace and World.
Hopkins-Kavanagh, K. (1989). Nurses networks: Obstacles and challenges. *Archives of Psychiatric Nursing, 3*(4), 226-233.
Horman, S. (1989). The role of social support on health throughout the lifecycle. *Health Education, 20*(4), 18-21.
House, J. S. (1981). Work stress and social support. Englewood Cliffs, NJ: Prentice Hall.
House, J. S., & Kahn, R. L. (1985). Measures and concepts of social support. In S. Cohen & S. L. Syme (Eds.), *Social support and health* (pp. 83-108). Orlando, FL: Academic Press.
House, J. S., Kessler, R. C., & Herzog, A. R. (1990). Age, socioeconomic status, and health. *Milbank Quarterly, 68*(3), 383-411.
House, J. S., Landis, K. R., & Umberson, D. (1988). Social relationships and health. *Science, 241,* 540-545.
House, J. S., Robbins, C., & Metzner, H. C. (1982). The association of social relationships and activities with mortality: Prospective evidence from the Tecumseh community health study. *American Journal of Epidemiology, 116,* 123-140.
House, J. S., Umberson, D., & Landis, K. (1988). Structures and processes of social support. *Annual Review of Sociology, 14,* 293-318.
Houston, B., & Vavak, C. (1991). Cynical hostility: Developmental factors, psychosocial correlates, and health behaviors. *Health Psychology, 10*(1), 9-17.
Hubbard, P., Muhlenkamp, P. A., & Brown, N. (1984). The relationship between social support and self-care practices. *Nursing Research, 33*(5), 266-270.
Ihlenfeld, J. T. (1991). Social support in student nurse clinical groups. *Nurse Educator, 16*(1), 15, 25, 29.
Ingersoll-Dayton, B., & Antonucci, T. C. (1988). Reciprocal and non-reciprocal social support: Contrasting sides of intimate relationships. *Journal of Gerontology, 43,* 565-573.
Israel, B., Schurman, S., & House, J. (1989). Active research on occupational stresses involving workers as researchers. *International Journal of Health Services, 8*(1), 135-155.
Jackson, B. B. (1985). Role of social resource variables upon life satisfaction in black climacteric hysterectomized women. *Nursing Papers, 17,* 4-22.
Jacobs, M., & Goodman, G. (1989). Psychology and self-help groups: Predictions on a partnership. *American Psychology, 44,* 536-545.
Jacobson, D. (1990). Stress and support in stepfamily formation: The cultural context of social support. In B. R. Sarason, I. G. Sarason, & G. R. Pierce (Eds.), *Social support: An interactional view* (pp. 199-218). New York: John Wiley.
Jacobson, D. E. (1986). Types and timing of social support. *Journal of Health and Social Behavior, 27,* 250-264.
Jacox, A. (1981). *Competing theories of science.* Paper presented at Forum on Doctoral Education in Nursing, Seattle, WA.
Jarvis, P. (1983). *Professional education.* London: Croom Helm.
Jeger, A. M., Slotnick, R. S., & Schure, M. (1982). Toward a self-help/professional collaborative perspective in mental health. In D. Biegel & A. J. Naparstek (Eds.), *Community support systems and mental health* (pp. 205-223). New York: Springer.

Jennings, B. (1990). Stress, locus of control, social support and psychological symptoms among head nurses. *Research in Nursing and Health, 13*, 393-401.

Jessop, D. J., & Stein, R. E. K. (1991). Who benefits from a pediatric home care program? *Pediatrics, 88*(3), 497-505.

Johnson, D. E. (1974). Development of theory: A requisite for nursing as a primary health profession. *Nursing Research, 23*, 372-377.

Johnson, D. E. (1980). The behavioral system model for nursing. In J. P. Riehl & C. Roy (Eds.), *Conceptual models for nursing practice* (2nd ed.). New York: Appleton-Century-Crofts.

Jones, W. H. (1985). The psychology of loneliness: Some personality issues in the study of social support. In I. G. Sarason & B. R. Sarason (Eds.), *Social support: Theory, research, application* (pp. 225-242). Dordrecht, The Netherlands: Martinus Nijhoff.

Jordan, P. (1985). Network structure, social support, and parent adaptation to the birth of a second child. In R. A. O'Brien (Ed.), *Social support and health: New directions for theory and research* (pp. 175-179). Rochester, NY: University of Rochester Press.

Jung, J. (1990). The role of reciprocity in social support. *Basic and Applied Social Psychology, 11*(3), 243-253.

Kahn, R. L., & Antonucci, T. C. (1980). Convoys over the life course: Attachment, roles and social support. In P. B. Baltes & O. Brim (Eds.), *Life span development and behavior* (pp. 253-286). New York: Academic Press.

Kaplan, B. H., Cassel, J. C., & Gore, S. (1977). Social support and health. *Medical Care, 15*(5), 47-58.

Kaplan, R. M., & Toshima, T. (1990). The functional effects of social relationships on chronic illnesses and disability. In B. R. Sarason, I. B. Sarason, & G. R. Pierce (Eds.), *Social support: An interactional view* (pp. 427-453). New York: John Wiley.

Kasl, S., & Wells, J. (1985). Social support and health in the middle years: Work and the family. In S. Cohen & S. L. Syme (Eds.), *Social support and health* (pp. 175-198). Orlando, FL: Academic Press.

Katz, A. H. (1981). Self-help and mutual aid: An emerging social movement. *Annual Review of Sociology, 7*, 129-155.

Katz, A. H. (1985). Where are self-help studies going? *Journal of Primary Prevention, 6*(2), 128-136.

Katz, A. H., & Bender, E. I. (1990). *Helping one another: Self-help groups in a changing world.* Oakland, CA: Third Party.

Katz, A. H., & Levin, L. S. (1980). Self-care is *not* a solipsistic trap: A reply to critics. *International Journal of Health Services, 10*(2), 329-336.

Kaufman, K. J. (1986). *Social-psychological influences on breast-feeding of preterm infants.* Unpublished doctoral dissertation, University of North Carolina, Chapel Hill.

Kaufman, K. J., & Hall, L. A. (1989). Influences of the social network on choice and duration of breast-feeding in mothers of preterm infants. *Research in Nursing and Health, 12*, 149-159.

Kelley, H. H. (1967). Attribution theory in social psychology. In D. Levine (Ed.), *Nebraska Symposium on Motivation, 1967* (pp. 192-240). Lincoln: University of Nebraska Press.

Kelly, K. M., Sautter, F., Tugrul, K., & Weaver, M. (1990). Fostering self-help on an in-patient unit. *Archives of Psychiatric Nursing, 4*(3), 161-165.

Kelly, R., Zyzanski, S., & Alemagne, S. (1991). Prediction of motivation and behavior change following health promotion: Role of health beliefs, social support and self-efficacy. *Social Science and Medicine, 32*(3), 311-320.

Kelner, M. J. (1986). Toronto: University of Toronto. Personal communication.

Kennedy, S., Kiecolt-Glaser, J., & Glaser, R. (1990). Social support, stress and the immune system. In B. R. Sarason, I. B. Sarason, & G. R. Pierce (Eds.), *Social support: An interactional view* (pp. 253-266). New York: John Wiley.

Kessler, R. C., McLeod, J. P., & Wethington, E., (1985). The costs of caring: A perspective on the relationship between sex and psychological distress. In I. B. Sarason & B. R. Sarason (Eds.), *Social support: Theory, research, application* (pp. 491-505). Dordrecht, The Netherlands: Martinus Nijhoff.

Kickbusch, I. (1986). Health promotion: A global perspective. *Canadian Journal of Public Health, 77*, 321-326.

Kiecolt-Glaser, J. K., Ricker, D., George, J., Messick, G., Speicher, C. E., Garner, W., & Glaser, R. (1984). Urinary cortisol levels, cellular immunocompletency, and loneliness in psychiatric inpatients. *Psychosomatic Medicine, 41*(1), 15-23.

Killien, M. G., & Shy, K. (1989). A randomized trial of electronic fetal monitoring in preterm labor: Mothers' views. *Birth, 16*(1), 7-12.

Kim, H. S. (1983a). Collaborative decision-making in nursing practice: A theoretical framework. In P. L. Chinn (Ed.), *Advances in nursing theory development* (pp. 271-283). Rockville, MD: Aspen.

Kim, H. S. (1983b). *The nature of theoretical thinking in nursing*. Norwalk, CT: Appleton-Century-Crofts.

King, H. (1991). A telephone reassurance service: A natural support system for the elderly. *Journal of Gerontological Social Work, 16*(1/2), 159-177.

King, I. M. (1971). *Toward a theory for nursing: General concepts of human behavior*. New York: John Wiley.

King, I. M. (1981). *A theory for nursing: Systems, concepts, process*. New York: John Wiley.

King, I. M. (1984). Philosophy of nursing education: A national survey. *Western Journal of Nursing Research, 6*(4), 387-402.

King, I. M. (1986). *Curriculum and instruction in nursing: Concepts and process*. Englewood Cliffs, NJ: Prentice Hall.

Kinoy, B. P. (1985). Self-help groups in the management of anorexia nervosa and bulemia: A theoretical base. *Transactional Analysis Journal, 15*(1), 73-78.

Kirgis, C., Godfrey, A., & NcNeal, C. (1991). Nurses' supportive acts for mother-preterm infant pairs. *Child Health Care, 20*(3), 144-149.

Kirk, J., & Miller, M. (1986). *Reliability and validity in qualitative research*. Beverly Hills, CA: Sage.

Kirschling, J. M., Tilden, V. P., & Butterfield, P. G. (1990). Social support: The experience of hospice family caregivers. *Hospice Journal, 6*(2), 75-93.

Klass, D., & Shinners, B. (1983). Professional roles in a self-help group for the bereaved. *Omega, 13*(4), 361-375.

Kliewer, W., Lepore, S. J., Broquet, A., & Zuba, L. (1990). Developmental and gender differences in anonymous support-seeking: Analysis of data from a community help line for children. *American Journal of Community Psychology, 18*(2), 333-339.

Kobasa, S. (1979). Stressful life events, personality and health: An inquiry into hardiness. *Journal of Personality and Social Psychology, 37*, 1-11.

Kobasa, S., Muddi, S., Puccetti, M., & Zola, M. (1985). Effectiveness of hardiness, exercise and social support as resources against illness. *Social Science and Medicine, 19*, 525-533.

Kuhn, T. S. (1970). *The structure of scientific revolutions.* Chicago: University of Chicago Press.

Kuhn, T. S. (1977). *The essential tension.* Chicago: University of Chicago Press.

Kurtz, L. F. (1984). Ideological differences between professionals and AA members. *Alcoholism Treatment Quarterly, 1*(2), 73-85.

Kurtz, L. F. (1990). The self-help movement: Review of the past decade of research. *Social Work with Groups, 13*(3), 101-115.

Kurtz, L. F., Mann, K. B., & Cambon, A. (1987). Linking between social workers and mental health mutual-aid groups. *Social Work and Health Care, 13*(1), 69-78.

La Gaipa, J. J. (1990). The negative effects of informal support systems. In S. Duck (Ed.), *Personal relationships and social support* (pp. 122-139). London: Sage.

Lakey, B., & Cassady, P. (1990). Cognitive processes in perceived social support. *Journal of Personality and Social Psychology, 59*(2), 337-343.

Lakey, B., & Heller, K. (1988). Social support from a friend, perceived support, and social problem solving. *American Journal of Community Psychology, 16*(6), 811-824.

Lambert, V. A., Lambert, C. E., Klipple, G. L., & Mewshaw, E. A. (1989). Social support, hardiness and psychological well-being in women with arthritis. *Image: Journal of Nursing Scholarship, 21*(3), 128-131.

Landerman, R., George, L., Campbell, R., & Blazer, D. (1989). Alternative models of the stress buffering hypothesis. *American Journal of Community Psychology, 17*(5), 625-642.

LaRocco, J. M., House, J. S., & French, J. R. (1980). Social support, occupational stress and health. *Journal of Health and Social Behavior, 21*, 202-218.

Larson, M. S. (1977). *The rise of professionalism.* Berkeley: University of California Press.

Laschinger, S. (1984). The relationship of social support to health in elderly people. *Western Journal of Nursing Research, 6*(3), 341-350.

Laura, R. S. (1985). The philosophical foundations of medical education. *Educational Philosophy and Theory, 17*(2), 29-41.

Lazarus, R. S., & Folkman, S. (1984). *Stress, appraisal and coping.* New York: Springer.

Leavy, R. (1982). Social support and psychological disorder: A review. *Journal of Community Psychology, 11*, 3-21.

LeBoterf, G. (1983). Reformulating participatory research. *Assignment Children, 63/64*, 167-192.

Lee, D. L. (1988). The support group training project. In B. H. Gottlieb (Ed.), *Marshaling social support: Formats, processes, and effects* (pp. 135-164). Newbury Park, CA: Sage.

Lefcourt, H. M., Martin, R. A., & Saleh, W. E. (1984). Locus of control and social support: Interactive moderators of stress. *Journal of Personality and Social Psychology, 47*, 378-389.

Lenrow, P. B., & Burch, R. W. (1981). Mutual aid and professional services: Opposing or complementary? In B. H. Gottlieb (Ed.), *Social networks and social support* (pp. 233-257). Beverly Hills, CA: Sage.

Lenrow, P. B., & Cowden, P. (1980). Human services, professionals and the paradox of institutional reform. *American Journal of Community Psychology, 8*(4), 463-484.

Lenz, E. R., Parks, P. L., Jenkins, L. S., & Jarrett, G. E. (1986). Life changes and instrumental support as predictors of illness in mothers of 6-month olds. *Research in Nursing and Health, 9*, 17-24.

Levine, M. E. (1971). Holistic nursing. *Nursing Clinics of North America, 6*, 253-264.

Levy, L. H. (1978). Self-help groups viewed by mental health professionals: A survey and comments. *American Journal of Community Psychology, 6*(4), 305-313.

Levy, L. H. (1983). Mutual support groups in Great Britain: A survey. *Social Science and Medicine, 17*(16), 1265-1275.

Levy, S. M., Herberman, R. B., Whiteside, T., Sonzo, K., Lee, J., & Kirkwood, J. (1990). Perceived social support and tumor estrogen/progesterone receptor status as predictors of natural killer cell activity in breast cancer patients. *Psychosomatic Medicine, 52*(1), 73-85.

Lieberman, M. A., & Bliwise, N. G. (1985). Comparisons among peer and professionally directed groups for the elderly: Implications for the development of self-help groups. *International Journal of Group Psychotherapy, 35*(2), 155-175.

Lieberman, M. A., & Mullan, T. J. (1978). Does help help? The adaptive consequences of obtaining help from professionals and social networks. *American Journal of Community Psychology, 6*, 499-517.

Lindeman, C. A. (1988). Patient education. *Annual Review of Nursing Research, 6*, 199-212.

Lindgren, C. L. (1990). Burnout and social support in family caregivers. *Western Journal of Nursing Research, 12*(4), 469-487.

Lindsey, A., Dodd, M. J., & Chen, S. (1985). Social support networks of Taiwanese cancer patients. *International Journal of Nursing Studies, 22*, 149-164.

Lindsey, E., & Attridge, C. (1989). Staff nurses' perceptions of support in an acute care workplace. *Canadian Journal of Nursing Research, 21*(5), 15-25.

Lindsey-Davis, L. (1990). Illness uncertainty, social support, and stress in recovering individuals and family caregivers. *Applied Nursing Research, 3*(2), 69-71.

Litwak, E. (1985). *Helping the elderly: The complementary roles of informal networks and formal systems.* New York: Guilford.

Lopata, H. Z., Jeinmann, G. D., & Baum, J. (1982). Loneliness: Antecedents and coping strategies in the lives of widows. In L. A. Peplau & D. Perlman (Eds.), *Loneliness: A sourcebook of current theory, research and therapy* (pp. 310-326). New York: John Wiley.

Lucas, C. (1985). Development and validation of the Perioperative Inventory of Supportive Behaviors. In R. A. O'Brien (Ed.), *Social support and health: New directions for theory and research* (pp. 149-153). Rochester, NY: University of Rochester Press.

MacCarthy, B. (1989). Needs for care among the relatives of long-term users of daycare. *Psychological Medicine, 19*, 725-736.

MacElveen-Hoehn, P., & Eyres, S. (1984). Social support and vulnerability in families and vulnerable infants. *Birth Defects: Original Article Series, 20*(5), 11-43.

Maclure, R. (1990). The challenge of participatory research and its implications for funding agencies. *International Journal of Sociology and Social Policy, 10*(3), 1-21.

Maguire, L. (1983). *Understanding social networks.* Beverly Hills, CA: Sage.

Maguire, L. (1991). *Social support systems in practice.* Silver Spring, MD: National Association of Social Workers Press.

Maida, C. A. (1985). Social support and learning in preventive health care. *Social Science and Medicine, 21*(3), 335-339.

Maier, S. F., Landenslager, M. L., & Ryan, S. M. (1985). Stressor controllability, immune function and endogenous opiates. In F. R. Brush & J. B. Overmier (Eds.), *Affect, conditioning and cognition: Essays on the determinants of behavior* (pp. 103-201). Hillsdale, NJ: Lawrence Erlbaum.

Malone, J. (1988). The social support-social dissupport continuum. *Journal of Psychosocial Nursing and Mental Health Services, 26*(12), 18-22.

Mansfield, P., Yu, L., McLeod, W., Vicary, J., & Packard, J. (1989). The job content index: A guide for improving the "fit" between nurses and their environment. *Journal of Advanced Nursing, 14*, 501-508.

Manthei, M. (1982). *A comparison of the effectiveness of professionals, non-professionals and self-help groups in teaching assertiveness.* Unpublished doctoral dissertation, University of Massachusetts. (Ann Arbor, MI: University Microfilms International, No. 8219825)

Marmar, C. R., Horowitz, M. J., Weiss, D. W., Wilner, N. R., & Kaltreider, N. B. (1988). A controlled trial of brief psychotherapy and mutual-help group treatment of conjugal bereavement. *American Journal of Psychiatry, 145*, 203-209.

Marques, C. C. (1983). *Behavior control self-help groups: Members' attitudes regarding health care professionals.* Unpublished doctoral dissertation, University of Arizona.

Marriner-Tomey, A. (1989). *Nursing theorists and their work.* St. Louis, MO: C. V. Mosby.

Marshall, J. R. (1989). Student attrition: Is lack of support a key? *Nursing Outlook, 37*(4), 176-178.

Maton, K. I. (1987). Patterns and psychological correlates of material support within a religious setting: The bidirectional support hypothesis. *American Journal of Community Psychology, 15*(2), 185-207.

Maton, K. I. (1988). Social support, organizational characteristics, psychological well-being and group appraisal in three self-help group populations. *American Journal of Community Psychology, 16*(1), 53-77.

McCain, N. L. (1985). A test of Cohen's developmental model for professional socialization with baccalaureate nursing students. *Journal of Nursing Education, 24*(5), 180-186.

McCloskey, J. (1990). Two requirements for job contentment: Autonomy and social integration. *Image: Journal of Nursing Scholarship, 22*(3), 140-143.

McConville, A. (1989). Setting up a parenting group. *Health Visitor, 62*(11), 338-339.

McCubbin, M. A. (1989). Family stress and family strengths: A comparison of single and two parent families with handicapped children. *Research in Nursing and Health, 12*, 101-110.

McCullough, M. A., Day, S., Herlihy, E., & Rapp, P. (1989). Using a multidisciplinary follow-up program to assist patient adjustment following temporal lobectomy. *Journal of Neuroscience Nursing, 21*(5), 295-304.

McGough, R. (1990). Assessing social support of people with AIDS. *Oncology Nursing Forum, 17*(1), 31-35.

McHaffie, H. E. (1989). Mothers of very low birth weight babies: Who supports them? *Midwifery, 5*, 113-121.

McKenna, L. S. (1985). Social network characteristics, perceived social support and level of psychological adaptation in battered women. In J. S. Norbeck (Ed.), *Proceedings of First International Nursing Research Conference on Social Support* (pp. 45-46). San Francisco: University of California.

McKinlay, J. (1982). Proletarianization of physicians. In C. Derber (Ed.), *Professionals as workers and mental labor in advanced capitalism* (pp. 39-69). Boston: G. K. Hall.
McNett, S. C. (1987). Social support, threat, and coping responses and effectiveness in the functionally disabled. *Nursing Research, 36*(2), 98-103.
Meagher, D., Gregor, F., & Stewart, M. (1987). Dyadic social support interventions for cardiac surgery patients: A Canadian approach. *Social Science and Medicine, 25*(7), 833-837.
Meleis, A. I. (1985). *Theoretical nursing: Development and progress* (1st ed.). Philadelphia: J. B. Lippincott.
Meleis, A. I. (1991). *Theoretical nursing: Development and progress* (2nd ed.). Philadelphia: J. B. Lippincott.
Melnyk, K. A. (1988). Barriers: A critical review of recent literature. *Nursing Research, 37*(4), 196-201.
Melucci, A. (1984). An end to social movements? Introductory paper to the sessions on "New movements and change in organizational forms." *Social Science Information, 23*(4), 819-835.
Melucci, A. (1985). The symbolic challenge of contemporary movements. *Social Research, 52*(4), 790-816.
Mercer, R. T., Hackley, K. C., & Bostrom, A. (1984). Social support of teenage mothers. *Birth Defects: Original Article Series, 20*(5), 245-290.
Mermelstein, R. J., Lichtenstein, E., & McIntyre, K. O. (1983). Partner support and relapse in smoking cessation programs. *Journal of Consulting and Clinical Psychology, 51*, 465-466.
Merton, R. K. (1968). *Social theory and social structure.* New York: Free Press.
Miller, A. (1985). The relationship between nursing theory and nursing practice. *Journal of Advanced Nursing, 10*, 417-424.
Miller, G. P. (1983). *Professionals' knowledge of, referrals to, utilization of, linkages with and attitudes toward self-help groups.* Unpublished doctoral dissertation, University of Michigan, Ann Arbor.
Miller, P., McMahon, M. A., & Garrett, M. J. (1989). A content analysis of life adjustments post infarction. *Western Journal of Nursing Research, 11*(5), 559-567.
Minkler, M. (1985). Social support and the health of the elderly. In S. Cohen & S. L. Syme (Eds.), *Social support and health* (pp. 199-218). Orlando, FL: Academic Press.
Minkler, M. (1986). The social component of health. *American Journal of Health Promotion, 1*(2), 23-38.
Mishel, M. H., & Braden, C. J. (1987). Uncertainty: A mediator between support and adjustment. *Western Journal of Nursing Research, 9*, 43-57.
Mitchell, J. C. (1969). *Social networks in urban situations.* Manchester, UK: Manchester University Press.
Mitchell, R. H., & Trickett, R. E. (1982). Social network resources and adaptation: A conceptual framework. In T. A. Wills (Ed.), *Basic processes in helping relationships* (pp. 213-232). New York: Academic Press.
Mohide, E., Pringle, D., Steiner, D., Gilbert, J., Muir, G., & Tew, M. (1990). A randomized trial of family caregiver support in the home management of dementia. *Journal of the American Geriatrics Society, 38*, 446-454.
Montgomery-Hunter, S., & Striden-Hall, S. (1989). The effect of an educational support program on dyspnea and the emotional status of COPD clients. *Rehabilitation Nursing, 14*(4), 200-202.

Morisky, D. E., DeMuth, N. M., Field-Fass, M., Green, L. W., & Levine, D. M. (1985). Evaluation of family health education to build social support for long-term control of high blood pressure. *Health Education Quarterly, 12*, 35-50.

Morisky, D. E., Levine, D. M., Green, L. W., Shapiro, S., Russell, P., & Smith, C. R. (1983). Five-year blood pressure control and mortality following health education for hypertensive patients. *American Journal of Public Health, 73*, 153-162.

Morse, J. M. (1989). *Qualitative nursing research: A contemporary dialogue*. Rockville, MD: Aspen.

Mowrer, O. H. (1960). *Learning theory and the symbolic processes*. New York: John Wiley.

Muhlenkamp, A. F., & Sayles, J. A. (1986). Self-esteem, social support and health practices. *Nursing Research, 35*(6), 334-338.

Murphy, S. A. (1987). Self-efficacy and social support: Mediators of stress on mental health following a natural disaster. *Western Journal of Nursing Research, 9*, 58-86.

Newcomb, M. (1990). Social support by many other names: Towards a unified conceptualization. *Journal of Social and Personal Relationships, 7*(4), 479-494.

Newman, M. A. (1983). The continuing revolution: A history of nursing science. In N. Chaska (Ed.), *The nursing profession: A time to speak* (pp. 385-393). Toronto: McGraw-Hill.

Norbeck, J. S. (1981). Social support: A model for clinical research and application. *Advances in Nursing Science, 7*, 43-59.

Norbeck, J. S. (1982). The use of social support in clinical practice. *Journal of Psychiatric and Mental Health Services, 20*(12), 22-29.

Norbeck, J. S. (1984). The Norbeck Social Support Questionnaire. *Birth Defects: Original Article Series, 20*(5), 45-55.

Norbeck, J. S. (1985a). International nursing research in social support: Background concepts and methodological issues. In *Proceedings of First International Nursing Conference on Social Support* (pp. 1-20). Tel Aviv.

Norbeck, J. S. (1985b). Measurement of social support: Recent strategies and continuing issues. In R. A. O'Brien (Ed.), *Social support and health: New directions for theory and research* (pp. 73-106). Rochester, NY: University of Rochester Press.

Norbeck, J. S. (1985c). Perceived job stress, job satisfaction and psychological symptoms in critical care nursing. *Research in Nursing and Health, 8*, 253-259.

Norbeck, J. S. (1985d). Types and sources of social support for managing job stress in critical care nursing. *Nursing Research, 34*(4), 225-230.

Norbeck, J. S. (1988a). Challenges in social support research. The Eighth Helen Nahm Research Lecture. University of California, San Francisco.

Norbeck, J. S. (1988b). Social support. *Annual Review of Nursing Research, 6*, 85-109.

Norbeck, J. S. (1991a). Contributions of nurses to social support research. Presentation to School of Nursing, Dalhousie University, Halifax, Nova Scotia, Canada.

Norbeck, J. S. (1991b). Social support needs of family caregivers of psychiatric patients from three age groups. *Nursing Research, 40*(4), 208-213.

Norbeck, J. S., & Anderson, N. J. (1989a). Life stress, social support, and anxiety in mid- and late-pregnancy among low income women. *Research in Nursing and Health, 12*, 281-287.

Norbeck, J. S., & Anderson, N. J. (1989b). Psychosocial predictors of pregnancy outcomes in low-income black, hispanic, and white women. *Nursing Research, 38*(4), 204-209.

Norbeck, J. S., Lindsey, A., & Carrieri, V. (1981). The development of an instrument to measure social support. *Nursing Research, 30*(4), 264-269.

Norbeck, J. S., Lindsey, A., & Carrieri, V. (1983). Further development of the Norbeck Social Support Questionnaire: Normative data and validity testing. *Nursing Research, 32*(1), 4-9.

Norbeck, J. S., & Sheiner, M. (1982). Sources of social support related to single parent functioning. *Research in Nursing and Health, 5,* 3-12.

Norbeck, J. S., & Tilden, V. P. (1983). Life stress, social support and emotional disequilibrium in complications of pregnancy: A prospective multivariate study. *Journal of Health and Social Behavior, 24,* 30-46.

Norbeck, J. S., & Tilden, V. P. (1988). International nursing research in social support: Theoretical and methodological issues. *Journal of Advanced Nursing, 13,* 173-178.

Northouse, L. L. (1988). Social support in patients' and husbands' adjustment to breast cancer. *Nursing Research, 37,* 91-97.

O'Brien, R. A. (1985). Social support and health maintenance during early bereavement. In R. A. O'Brien (Ed.), *Social support and health: New directions for theory development and research* (pp. 203-207). Rochester, NY: University of Rochester Press.

O'Leary, A. (1985). Self-efficacy and health. *Behavioral Research Therapy, 4,* 437-451.

O'Reilly, P. (1988). Methodological issues in social support and social network research. *Social Science and Medicine, 26*(8), 863-873.

Ockene, J. K., Benfari, R. C., Nuttall, R. L., Hurwitz, I., & Ockene, I. S. (1982). Relationship of psychosocial factors to smoking behavior change in an intervention program. *Preventive Medicine, 11,* 13-28.

Oehler, J. M., Peter, M. A., & Seyler, S. (1989). Support groups: Are they really helpful in dealing with NICU stress? *Neonatal Network, 8*(2), 21-25.

Offe, C. (1984). *Contradictions of the welfare state.* Cambridge: MIT Press.

Offe, C. (1985). New social movements: Challenging the boundaries of institutional politics. *Social Research, 52*(4), 817-868.

Ogus, L. (1990). Burnout and social support systems among ward nurses. *Issues in Mental Health Nursing, 11,* 261-281.

Okun, M. A., Sandler, I. N., & Baumann, D. J. (1988). Buffer and booster effects as event-support transactions. *American Journal of Community Psychology, 16,* 435-449.

Okun, M. D., Melichar, J. F., & Hill, M. D. (1990). Negative daily events, positive and negative social ties, and psychological distress among older adults. *The Gerontologist, 30*(2), 193-199.

Olds, D., Henderson, C., Tatelbaum, R., & Chamber, R. (1988). Improving the life course development of socially disadvantaged mothers: A randomized trial of nurse home visitation. *American Journal of Public Health, 78,* 1436-1445.

Olds, D., & Kitzman, H. (1990). Can home visitation improve the health of women and children at environmental risk? *Pediatrics, 86*(1), 108-116.

Olsen, O., Iversen, L., & Sabroe, S. (1991). Age and the operationalization of social support. *Social Science and Medicine, 32*(7), 767-771.

Orem, D. E. (1980). *Nursing: Concepts of practice* (2nd ed.). New York: McGraw-Hill.

Pagana, K. D. (1990). The relationship of hardiness and social support to student appraisal of stress in an initial clinical nursing situation. *Journal of Nursing Education, 29*(6), 255-261.

Palmblad, J. (1981). Stress and immunologic competence: Studies in man. In R. Ader (Ed.), *Psychoneuroimmunology* (pp. 229-257). New York: Academic Press.

Parmalee, P. A. (1983). Spouse versus other family caregivers: Psychological impact on impaired aged. *American Journal of Community Psychology, 11*(4), 337-349.

Parse, R. R. (1981). *Man-living-health: A theory of nursing*. New York: John Wiley.

Pasacreta, J., & Jacobsen, P. (1989). Addressing the need for staff support among nurses caring for the AIDS population. *Oncology Nursing Forum, 16*(5), 659-663.

Pasquarello, M. (1990). Developing, implementing and evaluating a stroke recovery group. *Rehabilitation Nursing, 15*(1), 26-29.

Pearlin, L. (1985). Social structure and processes of social support. In S. Cohen & S. L. Syme (Eds.), *Social support and health* (pp. 43-60). Orlando, FL: Academic Press.

Pearlin, L., Lieberman, M., Menaghan, E., & Mullan, J. (1981). The stress process. *Journal of Health and Social Behavior, 22*, 337-356.

Pender, N. J. (1987). *Health promotion in nursing practice.* Norwalk, CT: Appleton & Lange.

Pennebaker, J. W., Kiecolt-Glaser, J. K., & Glaser, R. (1988). Disclosure of traumas and immune function: Health implications for psychotherapy. *Journal of Consulting and Clinical Psychology, 56*, 239-245.

Perlman, D., & Fehr, B. (1987). The development of intimate relationships. In D. Perlman & S. Duck (Eds.), *Intimate relationships: Development, dynamics, and deterioration* (pp. 1-42). Newbury Park, CA: Sage.

Peters-Golden, H. (1982). Breast cancer: Varied perceptions of social support in the illness experience. *Social Science and Medicine, 23*(5), 483-491.

Peterson, L. (1990). Phone friend: A developmental description of needs expressed by child callers to a community telephone support system for children. *Journal of Applied Developmental Psychology, 11*(1), 105-122.

Pierce, G. R., Sarason, B. R., & Sarason, I. G. (1990). Integrating social support perspectives: Working models, personal relationships and situational factors. In S. Duck (Ed.), *Personal relationships and social support* (pp. 173-189). London: Sage.

Pierce, L., & Salter, J. (1988). Stroke support group a reality. *Rehabilitative Nursing, 13* (4), 189-190.

Pilisuk, M. (1982). Delivery of social support: The social inoculation. *American Journal of Orthopsychiatry, 52*(1), 20-31.

Pilisuk, M., & Minkler, M. (1985). Social support: Economic and political considerations. *Social Policy, 15*(3), 6-11.

Platt, C. (1990). An experiment in psychiatric community care in North Staffordshire: The experience of working with relatives of mentally ill people. *Journal of Advanced Nursing, 15*, 1315-1318.

Pohl, J., & Fuller, S. (1980). Perceived choice, social interaction and dimensions of morale of residents in a home for the aged. *Research in Nursing and Health, 3*, 147-157.

Polit, D. F., & Hungler, B. P. (1991). *Nursing research: Principles and methods* (4th ed.). Philadelphia: J. B. Lippincott.

Popiel, D. A., & Susskind, E. C. (1985). The impact of rape: Social support as a moderator of stress. *American Journal of Community Psychology, 13*(6), 645-676.

Popkewitz, T. S. (1984). *Paradigm and ideology in educational research.* London: Falmer.

Potter, J., & Wetherell, M. (1989). *Discourse and social psychology: Beyond attitudes and behaviors.* Newbury Park, CA: Sage.

Powell, D. R. (1988). Support groups for low-income mothers: Design considerations and patterns of participation. In B. H. Gottlieb (Ed.), *Marshalling social support: Formats, processes, and effects* (pp. 111-134). Newbury Park, CA: Sage.

Powell, T. J., & Cameron, M. J. (1991). Self-help research and the public mental health system. *American Journal of Community Psychology, 19*(5), 797-805.

Powers, B. (1985). Social networks of elderly institutionalized people. In R. A. O'Brien (Ed.), *Social support and health: New directions for theory and research* (pp. 190-193). Rochester, NY: University of Rochester Press.

Pridham, K. F. (1984). Information needs and problem solving behavior of parents of infants. *Birth Defects: Original Article Series, 20*(5), 125-165.

Primono, J., Yates, B. C., & Woods, N. F. (1990). Social support for women during chronic illness: The relationship among sources and types of adjustment. *Research in Nursing and Health, 13*, 153-161.

Printz-Fedderson, U. (1990). Group process effect on caregiver burden. *Journal of Neuroscience Nursing, 22*(3), 164-168.

Procidano, M. E., & Heller, K. I. (1983). Measures of perceived social support from friends and family: Three validation studies. *American Journal of Community Psychology, 11*, 1-24.

Pugliesi, K. (1989). Social support and self-esteem as intervening variables in the relationship between social roles and women's well-being. *Community Mental Health Journal, 25*(2), 87-100.

Puskar, K., Lamb, J., & Martsolf, D. (1990). The role of the psychiatric/mental health nurse clinical specialist in an adolescent coping skills group. *Journal of Child and Adolescent Psychiatric and Mental Health Nursing, 3*(2), 47-51.

Quittner, A. L., Glueckouf, R. L., & Jackson, D. N. (1990). Chronic parenting stress: Moderating versus mediating effects of social support. *Journal of Personality and Social Psychology, 59*(6), 1266-1278.

Raatikainen, R. (1991). Social support, participation and collaboration of relatives in domiciliary care. *International Journal of Nursing Studies, 28*(4), 377-386.

Ramphele, M. (1990). Participatory research: The myths and realities. *Social Dynamics, 16*(2), 1-15.

Rappaport, J. (1985). The power of empowerment language. *Social Policy, 16*(2), 15-21.

Rawls, J. (1971). *A theory of justice.* Cambridge, MA: Harvard University Press.

Reed, P. G. (1986). A model for constructing a conceptual framework for education in the clinical specialty. *Journal of Nursing Education, 25*(7), 295-299.

Rehr, H., & Rosenberg, G. (1991). Social-health care: Problems and predictions. *Journal of Gerontological Social Work, 16*(1/2), 97-120.

Reiss, H. T. (1984). Social interaction and well-being. In S. Duck (Ed.), *Personal relationships: Repairing personal relationships* (pp. 21-45). London: Academic Press.

Revicki, D. A., & May, H. J. (1989). Organizational characteristics, occupational stress, and mental health in nurses. *Behavioral Medicine, 15*(1), 30-36.

Rheume, A., & Gooding, B. (1991). Social support, coping strategies and long-term adaptation to ostomy among self-help group members. *Journal of Enterostomy Therapy, 18*, 11-15.

Ribble, D. (1989). Psychological support groups for people with HIV infection and AIDS. *Holistic Nursing Practice, 3*(4), 52-62.

Rich, O. J. (1978). The sociogram: A tool for depicting support in pregnancy. *Maternal-Child Nursing Journal, 7*, 1-9.

Richardson, P. (1987). Women's important relationships during pregnancy and the preterm labor event. *Western Journal of Nursing Research, 9*(2), 203-222.

Riehl, J. P. (1980). The Riehl interaction model. In J. P. Riehl & C. Roy (Eds.), *Conceptual models for nursing practice* (pp. 350-356). New York: Appleton-Century-Crofts.

Riffle, K. L. (1989). Stress: Nurses dealing with family members. *Journal of Gerontological Nursing, 15*(7), 18-25.

Riffle, K. L., Yoho, J., & Sams, J. (1989). Health-promoting behaviors, perceived social support, and self-reported health of Appalachian elderly. *Public Health Nursing, 6*(4), 204-211.

Riley, D., & Eckenrode, J. (1986). Social ties: Subgroup differences in costs and benefits. *Journal of Personality and Social Psychology, 51*(4), 770-778.

Robinson, K. (1990). The relationship between social skills, social support, self-esteem, and burden in adult caregivers. *Journal of Advanced Nursing, 15*, 788-795.

Rodin, J., & Ickovics, J. (1990). Women's health: Review and research agenda as we approach the 21st century. *American Psychologist, 45*(9), 1018-1034.

Romeder, J. M. (1982). *Self-help groups in Canada.* Ottawa, Ontario, Canada: Health and Welfare Canada.

Rook, K. S. (1984). Promoting social bonding strategies for helping the lonely and socially isolated. *American Psychology, 39*, 1389-1407.

Rook, K. S. (1985). The functions of social bonds: Perspectives from research on social support, loneliness and social isolation. In I. G. Sarason & B. R. Sarason (Eds.), *Social support: Theory, research, and applications* (pp. 243-286). Dordrecht, The Netherlands: Martinus Nijhoff.

Rook, K. S. (1987). Reciprocity of social exchange and social satisfaction among older women. *Journal of Personality and Social Psychology, 52*, 145-154.

Rook, K. S. (1990). Parallels in the study of social support and social strain. *Journal of Social and Clinical Psychology, 9*(1), 118-132.

Rook, K. S., Catalano, R., & Dooley, D. (1989). The timing of major life events: Effects of departing from the social clock. *American Journal of Community Psychology, 17*(2), 233-258.

Rook, K. S., & Dooley, D. (1985). Applying social support research: Theoretical problems and future directions. *Journal of Social Issues, 41*, 5-28.

Rook, K. S., & Pietromonaco, P. (1987). Close relationships: Ties that heal or ties that bind. In D. Perlman & W. Jones (Eds.), *Advances in personal relationships* (pp. 1-35). Greenwich, CT: JAI Press.

Rootman, I. (1989). *Knowledge of health promotion: A summary of Canadian literature reviews.* Ottawa, Ontario, Canada: Health and Welfare Canada.

Rounds, K. A., Galinsky, M. J., & Stevens, L. S. (1991). Linking people with AIDS in rural communities: The telephone group. *Social Work, 36*(1), 13-17.

Roy, C. (1984). *Introduction to nursing: An adaptation model* (2nd ed.). Englewood Cliffs, NJ: Prentice Hall.

Roy, C., & Roberts, S. L. (1981). *Theory construction in nursing: An adaptation model.* Englewood Cliffs, NJ: Prentice Hall.

Rueschemeyer, D. (1983). Professional autonomy and the social control of expertise. In R. Dingwall & P. Lewis (Eds.), *The sociology of the professions* (pp. 38-58). New York: St. Martin's.

Rutledge, D. N. (1987). Factors related to women's practice of breast self-examination. *Nursing Research, 36*, 117-121.

Ryan, J. M. (1985). *Models of help preferred by nurses and mutual aid organizations*. Unpublished doctoral dissertation, Boston University. (University Microfilms, No. 8524195)

Ryan, M., & Austin, A. (1989). Social supports and social networks in the aged. *Image: Journal of Nursing Scholarship, 21*(3), 176-180.

Sabo, K., Kraay, C., & Rudy, E. (1989). ICU family support group sessions: Family members' perceived benefits. *Applied Nursing Research, 2*, 82-89.

Sanders, G. S. (1982). Social comparison and perceptions of health and illness. In G. S. Sanders & J. Suls (Eds.), *Social psychology of health and illness* (pp. 129-157). Hillsdale, NJ: Lawrence Erlbaum.

Sandler, I. M., & Barrera, M., Jr. (1984). Toward a multimethod approach to assessing the effects of social support. *American Journal of Community Psychology, 12*, 3-52.

Sandler, I. M., Gersten, J. C., Reynolds, K., Kallgren, C. A., & Ramirez, R. (1988). Using theory and data to plan support interventions: Design of a program for bereaved children. In B. H. Gottlieb (Ed.), *Marshaling social support: Formats, processes, and effects* (pp. 53-84). Newbury Park, CA: Sage.

Sanfilippo, J., Galbraith, E., & Yussman, M. (1989). In-office infertility support group. *Obstetrics and Gynecology, 74*(3), 405-407.

Santora, D. (1983). Conceptual frameworks of undergraduate and graduate nursing programs. In N. Chaska (Ed.), *The nursing profession: A time to speak* (pp. 101-110). Toronto, Ontario, Canada: McGraw-Hill.

Sarason, B. R., Sarason, I. G., Hacker, T. A., & Basham, R. B. (1985). Concomitants of social support: Social skills, physical attractiveness and gender. *Journal of Personality and Social Psychology, 49*, 469-480.

Sarason, B. R., Sarason, I. G., & Pierce, G. R. (1990). *Social support: An interactional view*. New York: John Wiley.

Sarason, I. G., Levine, H., Basham, R., & Sarason, B. R. (1983). Assessing social support: The social support questionnaire. *Journal of Personality and Social Psychology, 44*, 127-139.

Sarason, I. G., & Sarason, B. R. (Eds.). (1985). *Social support: Theory, research, and application*. Dordrecht, The Netherlands: Martinus Nijhoff.

Saunders, J. M., & McCorkle, R. (1987). Social support and coping with lung cancer. *Western Journal of Nursing Research, 9*, 29-42.

Schaefer, C., Coyne, J. C., & Lazarus, R. S. (1982). The health related functions of social support. *Journal of Behavioral Medicine, 4*, 381-406.

Schank, M. J., & Long, M. A. (1989). Maintaining health and independence. *Journal of Gerontological Nursing, 15*(6), 8-11.

Schmitt, M. (1985). Summary and conclusions. In R. A. O'Brien (Ed.), *Social support and health: New directions for theory and research* (pp. 229-231). Rochester, NY: University of Rochester Press.

Schon, D. A. (1983). *The reflective practitioner: How professionals think in action*. New York: Basic Books.

Schon, D. A. (1987). *Educating the reflective practitioner*. San Francisco: Jossey-Bass.

Schulz, R., & Rau, M. (1985). Social support through the life course. In S. Cohen & S. L. Syme (Eds.), *Social support and health* (pp. 129-150). Orlando, FL: Academic Press.

Schuster, T., Kessler, R., & Aseltin, R. (1990). Supportive interactions, negative interactions and depressed mood. *American Journal of Community Psychology, 18*(3), 423-438.

Schwarzer, R., & Leppin, A. (1989). Social support and health: A meta-analysis. *Psychology and Health, 3,* 1-15.

Seeman, T. E., & Berkman, L. F. (1988). Structural characteristics with social networks and their relationship with social support in the elderly: Who provides support. *Social Science and Medicine, 26,* 737-749.

Selenkow, I. (1990). Enhancing coping strategies of PWA's in the home: Community health nursing implications. *AIDS Patient Care 4*(2), 42-44.

Sexton, D., & Stephen, S. (1991). Postpartum mothers' perceptions of nursing interventions for perinatal grief. *Neonatal Network, 9*(5), 47-51.

Sexton, M., Bross, D., Hebel, J. R., Schumann, B. C., Gerace, T., Lasser, N., & Wright, N. (in press). Risk factor changes in wives with husbands at high risk of CHD: The spin-off effect. *Journal of Behavioral Medicine.*

Shah, C. (1987). The health of children of low income families. *Canadian Medical Association Journal, 137,* 485-490.

Shinn, M., Lehmann, S., & Wong, N. W. (1984). Social interaction and social support. *Journal of Social Issues, 40*(4), 55-76.

Shumaker, S., & Brownell, A. (1984). Toward a theory of social support: Closing conceptual gaps. *Journal of Social Issues, 40*(4), 11-36.

Shumaker, S., & Hill, D. (1991). Gender differences in social support and physical health. *Health Psychology, 10*(2), 102-111.

Silver, R. C., Wortman, C. B., & Crofton, C. (1990). The role of coping in support provision: The self-presentational dilemma of victims of life crises. In B. R. Sarason, I. G. Sarason, & G. R. Pierce (Eds.), *Social support: An interactional view* (pp. 397-426). New York: John Wiley.

Silverman, P. (1980). *Mutual help groups: Organization and development.* Beverly Hills, CA: Sage.

Simpson, T. (1991). The family as a source of support for the critically ill adult. *AACN Clinical Issues in Critical Care Nursing, 2*(2), 229-235.

Singh, A., & Pandey, J. (1990). Social support as a moderator of the relationship between poverty and coping behaviors. *Journal of Social Psychology, 130*(4), 533-541.

Sirles, A., & Selleck, C. (1989). Cardiac disease and the family: Impact, assessment, and implications. *Journal of Cardiovascular Nursing, 3,* 23-32.

Skiles, L., & Hinson, B. (1989). Occupational burnout among correctional health workers. *AAOHN (American Association of Occupational Health Nurse Journal), 37*(9), 374-378.

Smith, D. H., & Pillemer, K. (1983). Self-help groups as social movement organizations: Social structure and social change. *Research in Social Movements, Conflicts and Change, 5,* 203-233.

Smith, J. A. (1981). The idea of health: A philosophical inquiry. *Advances in Nursing Science, 3,* 43-50.

Solomon, G. F. (1981). Emotional and personality factors in the onset and course of autoimmune disease, particularly rheumatoid arthritis. In R. Ader (Ed.), *Psychoneuroimmunology* (pp. 159-182). New York: Academic Press.

Solomon, G. F. (1987). Psychoneuroimmunology: Interactions between central nervous system and immune system. *Journal of Neurological Science Research, 18,* 1-9.

Solomon, G. F., & Amkraut, A. A. (1981). Psychoneuroendocrinological effects on the immune response. *Annual Review of Microbiology, 35,* 155-184.

Solomon, Z., Waysman, M., & Mikulincer, M. (1990). Family functioning, perceived social support, and combat-related psychopathology: The moderating role of loneliness. *Journal of Social and Clinical Psychology, 9*(4), 456-472.

Sorensen, G., & Verbrugge, L. M. (1987). Women, work, and health. *Annual Review of Public Health, 8*, 235-251.

Stanton, M. (1980). Nursing theories and the nursing process. In R. George (Ed.), *Nursing theories: The base for professional nursing practice: The nursing theories conference group* (pp. 319-337). Englewood Cliffs, NJ: Prentice Hall.

Stark, J. S., Lowther, M. N. A., Hagerty, B. M., & Orczyk, C. (1986). A conceptual framework for the study of preservice professional programs in colleges and universities. *Journal of Higher Education, 57*(3), 231-258.

Stein, C. H. (1991). Peer support telephone dyads for elderly women: The wrong intervention or the wrong research? *American Journal of Community Psychology, 19*(1), 91-98.

Sterling, Y. M. (1990). Resource needs of mothers managing chronically ill infants at home. *Neonatal Network, 9*(1), 55-59.

Stevens, B. J. (1984). *Nursing theory: Analysis, application, evaluation.* Boston: Little, Brown.

Stevens, P. E. (1989). A critical social reconceptualization of environment in nursing: Implications for methodology. *Advances in Nursing Science, 11*(4), 56-68.

Stewart, M. J. (1988). Curricular content of Canadian university schools of nursing on lay support groups. *Canadian Journal of Nursing Research, 20*(4), 59-72.

Stewart, M. J. (1989a). Nurses' preparedness for health promotion through linkage with mutual-aid self-help groups. *Canadian Journal of Public Health, 80*(2), 110-114.

Stewart, M. J. (1989b). Social support: Diverse theoretical perspectives. *Social Science and Medicine, 28*(12), 1275-1282.

Stewart, M. J. (1989c). Social support instruments created by nurse investigators. *Nursing Research, 38*(5), 268-275.

Stewart, M. J. (1989d). Social support intervention studies: A review and prospectus of nursing contributions. *International Journal of Nursing Studies, 26*(2), 93-114.

Stewart, M. J. (1989e). Target populations of nursing research on social support. *International Journal of Nursing Studies, 26*(2), 115-129.

Stewart, M. J. (1990a). Access to health care for economically disadvantaged Canadians: A model. *Canadian Journal of Public Health, 81*(6), 450-455.

Stewart, M. J. (1990b). Expanding theoretical conceptualizations of mutual-aid self-help groups. *Social Science and Medicine, 31*(9), 1057-1066.

Stewart, M. J. (1990c). From provider to partner: A conceptual framework for nursing education based on primary health care premises. *Advances in Nursing Science, 12*(2), 9-27.

Stewart, M. J. (1990d). Professional interface with mutual aid self-help groups: A review. *Social Science and Medicine, 31*(10), 1143-1158.

Stewart, M. J. (1992). *Occupational support, stressors and satisfaction experienced by community health nurses.* Manuscript submitted for publication.

Stewart, M. J., & Gregor, F. (1984). Early discharge and return to work following myocardial infarction. *Social Science and Medicine, 18*(12), 1027-1036.

Stroebe, M., & Stroebe, W. (1983). Who suffers more? Sex differences in health risks of the widowed. *Psychology Bulletin, 93*, 279-301.

Stuart, R., & Mitchell, C. (1978). Self-help weight control groups: A professional and a consumer perspective. *Psychiatric Clinics of North America, 1*(3), 697-711.

Styles, M. M. (1982). *On nursing: Toward a new endowment*. St. Louis, MO: C. V. Mosby.

Sullivan, W. P., & Poertner, J. (1989). Social support and life stress: A mental health consumer's perspective. *Community Mental Health Journal, 25*(1), 21-32.

Suls, J. M. (1977). Social comparison theory and research. In J. M. Suls & R. E. Miller (Eds.), *Social comparison processes: Theoretical and empirical perspectives* (pp. 1-19). New York: Hemisphere.

Susskind, E. L., & Klein, D. C. (1985). *Community research methods, paradigms and applications*. New York: Praeger Special Studies.

Swanson, K. M. (1991). Empirical development of a middle-range theory of caring. *Nursing Research, 40*(3), 161-166.

Syme, S. L. (1987). Social determinants of disease. *Annals of Clinical Research, 19*(2), 144-152.

Tardy, C. H. (1985). Social support measurement. *American Journal of Community Psychology, 13*(2), 187-202.

Taylor, S. E. (1983). Adjustment to threatening events: A theory of cognitive adaptation. *American Psychology, 11*, 1161-1173.

Taylor, S. E., Falke, R. L., Mazel, R. M., & Hilsberg, B. L. (1988). Sources of satisfaction and dissatisfaction among members of cancer support groups. In B. H. Gottlieb (Ed.), *Marshalling social support: Formats, processes, and effects* (pp. 187-208). Newbury Park, CA: Sage.

Teplitz, L., Egenes, K., & Brask, L. (1990). Life after sudden death: The development of a support group for automatic implantable cardioverter-defibrillator patients. *Journal of Cardiovascular Nursing, 4*(12), 20-32.

Thibodeau, J. A. (1983). *Nursing models: Analysis and evaluation*. Monterey, CA: Wadsworth.

Thoits, P. A. (1982). Conceptual, methodological and theoretical problems in social support as a buffer against life stress. *Journal of Health and Social Behavior, 23*, 145-159.

Thoits, P. A. (1983). Dimensions of life events that influence psychological distress: An evaluation and synthesis of the literature. In H. B. Kaplan (Ed.), *Psychosocial stress: Trends in theory and research* (pp. 33-104). New York: Academic Press.

Thoits, P. A. (1986). Social support as coping assistance. *Journal of Consulting and Clinical Psychology, 54*(4), 416-423.

Thompson, D. R. (1989). A randomized controlled trial of in-hospital nursing support for first-time myocardial infarction patients and their partners: Effects on anxiety and depression. *Journal of Advanced Nursing, 14*, 291-297.

Thompson, D. R., & Cordle, C. (1988). Support of wives of myocardial patients. *Journal of Advanced Nursing, 13*, 223-228.

Thompson, L. W., Gallagher, D., Neis, G., & Epstein, D. (1983). Evaluation of the effectiveness of professionals and non-professionals as instructors of "Coping with Depression" classes for elders. *The Gerontologist, 23*, 390-396.

Tilburg, T., Sonderen, E., & Ormel, J. (1991). The measurement of reciprocity in ego-centered networks of personal relationships: A comparison of various indices. *Social Psychology Quarterly, 54*(1), 54-66.

Tilden, V. P. (1985a). Cost and conflict: The darker side of social support. In R. A. O'Brien (Ed.), *Social support and health: New directions for theory and research* (pp. 154-158). Rochester, NY: University of Rochester Press.

Tilden, V. P. (1985b). *Implications of social support theory for nursing education.* Paper presented at International Council of Nurses 18th Quadrennial Congress, Tel Aviv, Israel.

Tilden, V. P. (1985c). Issues of conceptualization and measurement of social support in the construction of nursing theory. *Research in Nursing and Health, 8,* 199-206.

Tilden, V. P. (1988). *The Tilden Interpersonal Relationship Inventory: A summary.* Unpublished manuscript, Oregon Health Sciences University.

Tilden, V. P., & Galyen, R. D. (1987). Cost and conflict: The darker side of social support. *Western Journal of Nursing Research, 9*(1), 9-18.

Tilden, V. P., Nelson, C. A., & May, B. A. (1990). The IPR Inventory: Development and psychometric characteristics. *Nursing Research, 39*(6), 337-343.

Tilden, V. P., & Weinert, C. (1987). Social support and the chronically ill individual. *Nursing Clinics of North America, 22*(3), 613-620.

Todres, R. (1982). Professional attitudes, awareness and use of self-help groups. *Prevention in the Human Services, 1,* 91-98.

Tolsdorf, C. (1976). Social networks, support, and coping. *Family Process, 15,* 407-417.

Toro, P. A. (1986). A comparison of natural and professional help. *American Journal of Community Psychology, 14*(2), 140-159.

Toro, P. A., Zimmerman, M. A., Seidman, L., Reischl, T. M., Rappaport, J., Luke, D. A., & Roberts, L. J. (1988). Professionals in mutual help groups: Impact on social climate and members' behavior. *Journal of Consulting and Clinical Psychology, 56,* 631-632.

Torres, G. (1986). *Theoretical foundations of nursing.* Norwalk, CT: Appleton-Century-Crofts.

Toseland, R. W. (1990). Long-term effectiveness of peer-led and professionally led support groups for caregivers. *Social Service Review, 64*(2), 301-327.

Toseland, R. W., & Hacker, L. (1982). Self-help groups and professional involvement. *Social Work, 27*(6), 341-347.

Toseland, R. W., & Hacker, L. (1985). Social workers: Use of self-help groups as a resource for clients. *Social Work, 30*(3), 232-237.

Toseland, R. W., Rossiter, C. T., & Labrecque, M. (1989). The effectiveness of three group intervention strategies to support family caregivers. *American Journal of Orthopsychiatry, 59*(3), 420-429.

Toseland, R. W., Rossiter, C. M., Peak, T., & Hill, P. (1990). Therapeutic processes in peer led and professionally led support groups for caregivers. *International Journal of Group Psychotherapy, 40*(3), 279-303.

Touraine, A. (1985). An introduction to the study of social movements. *Social Research, 52*(4), 749-787.

Tracey, T. J., & Toro, P. (1989). Natural and professional help: A process analysis. *American Journal of Community Psychology, 17*(4), 443-458.

Traunstein, D. M. (1984). From mutual-aid self-help to professional service. *Social Casework, 65*(10), 622-627.

Travelbee, J. (1971). *Interpersonal aspects of nursing* (2nd ed.). Philadelphia: F. A. Davis.

Tucker, M., & Johnson, O. (1989). Competence promoting versus competence inhibiting social support for mentally retarded mothers. *Pediatrics, 48*(2), 95-107.

Tulman, L., & Fawcett, J. (1990). Functional status during pregnancy and the postpartum: A framework for practice. *Image: Journal of Nursing Scholarship, 22*(3), 191-194.

Unger, D. G., & Wandersman, L. P. (1985). Social support and adolescent mothers: Action research contributions to theory and application. *Journal of Social Issues, 41*(1), 29-45.

Vachon, M. L. S., Lyall, W. A. L., Rogers, J., Freedman-Letofsky, K., & Freeman, S. J. J. (1980). A controlled study of self-help intervention for widows. *American Journal of Psychiatry, 137*, 1380-1384.

Vachon, M. L. S., Rogers, J., Lyall, W. A. L., Lancee, W. J., Sheldon, A. R, & Freeman, S. J. J. (1982). Predictors and correlates of adaptation to conjugal bereavement. *American Journal of Psychiatry, 139*, 998-1002.

Vance, C. (1990). Is there a mentor in your career future? *Imprint, 36*(5), 41-42.

Vaux, A. (1989). *Social support: Theory, research, and intervention*. New York: Praeger.

Vaux, A. (1990). An ecological approach to understanding and facilitating social support. *Journal of Social and Personal Relationships, 7*(4), 507-518.

Vaux, A., & Athanassopulou, M. (1987). Social support appraisals and network resources. *Journal of Community Psychology, 15*, 537-555.

Vaux, A., & Harrison, D. (1985). Support network characteristics associated with support satisfaction and perceived support. *American Journal of Community Psychology, 13*(3), 245-267.

Ventura, J. N. (1982). Parent coping behaviors, parent functioning and infant temperament characteristics. *Nursing Research, 31*, 269-273.

Walker, K. N., MacBride, A., & Vachon, M. L. (1977). Social support networks and the crisis of bereavement. *Social Science and Medicine, 11*, 35-41.

Wallston, B. S., Alagna, S. W., & DeVellis, B. M. (1983). Social support and physical health. *Health Psychology, 2*(4), 367-391.

Ward, R. A. (1985). Informal networks and well-being in later life: A research agenda. *The Gerontologist, 25*(1), 55-61.

Warner, M. (1981). The rise of community participation: Its impact on health professionals and the health bureaucracy. In D. Coburn, C. D'Arcy, P. New, & G. Torrance (Eds.), *Health and Canadian society* (pp. 354-368). Don Mills, Ontario, Canada: Fitzhenry & Whiteside.

Watson, J. (1979). *Nursing: The philosophy and science of caring*. Boston: Little, Brown.

Watson, J. (1985). *Nursing: Human science and human care*. Norwalk, CT: Appleton-Century-Crofts.

Webb, C., & Wilson-Barnett, J. (1983). Hysterectomy: A study in coping with recovery. *Journal of Advanced Nursing, 8*, 311-319.

Weinert, C. (1987). A social support measure: PRQ 85. *Nursing Research, 36*(5), 273-277.

Weinert, C., & Brandt, P. A. (1987). Measuring social support with the Personal Resource Questionnaire. *Western Journal of Nursing Research, 9*(4), 589-602.

Weinert, C., & Tilden, V. P. (1990). Measures of social support: Assessment of validity. *Nursing Research, 39*(4), 212-216.

Weiss, R. (1974). The provisions of social relationships. In Z. Rubin (Ed.), *Doing unto others* (pp. 17-26). Englewood Cliffs, NJ: Prentice Hall.

Wellman, B. (1981). Applying network analysis to the study of support. In B. H. Gottlieb (Ed.), *Social networks in social support* (pp. 171-200). Beverly Hills, CA: Sage.

Wellman, B. (1982). Studying personal communities. In P. V. Marsden & N. Lin (Eds.), *Social structure and network analysis* (pp. 61-80). Beverly Hills, CA: Sage.

Wellman, B. (1985). From social support to social network. In I. G. Sarason & B. R. Sarason (Eds.), *Social support: Theory, research and applications* (pp. 205-222). Dordrecht, The Netherlands: Martinus Nijhoff.

Wells, J. A. (1989). The role of social support in creative coping. *Journal of Comparative Sociology and Religion, 15-16,* 42-45.

Wethington, E., & Kessler, R. C. (1986). Perceived support, received support and adjustment to stressful life events. *Journal of Health and Social Behavior, 27*(1), 78-89.

Wheeler, S., & Limbo, R. (1990). Blueprint for a perinatal bereavement support group. *Pediatric Nursing, 16*(4), 341-344, 377.

Whittaker, J., & Garbarino, J. (1983). *Social support networks: Informal helping in the human services.* New York: Aldine.

Wiggins, N. (1989). Education and support for the newly diagnosed cardiac family: A vital link in rehabilitation. *Journal of Advanced Nursing, 14*(1), 63-67.

Wilcox, B. L., & Birkel, R. C. (1983). Social networks and the help-seeking process. In A. Nadler, J. D. Fisher, & B. M. DePaulo (Eds.), *New directions in helping: Vol. 3* (pp. 235-252). New York: Academic Press.

Wilcox, B. L., & Vernberg, E. (1985). Conceptual and theoretical dilemmas facing social support research. In I. G. Sarason & B. R. Sarason (Eds.), *Social support: Theory, research and application* (pp. 3-20). Dordrecht, The Netherlands: Martinus Nijhoff.

Wills, T. A. (1983). Social comparison in coping and help-seeking. In B. M. DePaulo, A. Nadler, & J. D. Fisher (Eds.), *New directions in helping: Vol. 2* (pp. 109-141). New York: Academic Press.

Wills, T. A. (1985). Supportive functions of interpersonal relationships. In S. Cohen & S. L. Syme (Eds.), *Social support and health* (pp. 61-82). Orlando, FL: Academic Press.

Wilson, H. S. (1985). *Research in nursing.* Menlo Park, CA: Addison-Wesley.

Wodarski, J. S. (1981). Treatment of parents who abuse their children: A literature review and implications for professionals. *Child Abuse and Neglect, 5,* 351-360.

Wood, J. V., Taylor, S. E., & Lichtman, R. R. (1985). Social comparison in adjustment to breast cancer. *Journal of Personality and Social Psychology, 49,* 1169-1183.

Woods, N. F., & Catanzaro, M. (1988). *Nursing research: Theory and practice.* St. Louis, MO: C. V. Mosby.

Woods, N. F., & Earp, J. L. (1978). Women with cured breast cancer. *Nursing Research, 27,* 279-285.

World Health Organization. (1978). *Report of the international conference on primary health care in Alma Ata, USSR.* Geneva, Switzerland: Author.

World Health Organization. (1984). *Health promotion: A discussion document on the concepts and principles.* Copenhagen: World Health Organization Regional Office for Europe.

World Health Organization. (1985). *A guide to curriculum review for basic nursing education: Orientation to primary health care and community health.* Geneva, Switzerland: Author.

World Health Organization and International Council of Nurses. (1987). Regulatory mechanisms for nursing training and practice: Meeting primary health care needs: Conclusion and recommendations of a WHO study group. *International Nursing Review, 34*(2), 52-54.

Wortman, C. B. (1984). Social support and cancer: Conceptual and methodologic issues. *Cancer, 53,* 2339-2360.

Wortman, C. B., & Conway, T. L. (1985). The role of social support in adaptation and recovery from physical illness. In S. Cohen & S. L. Syme (Eds.), *Social support and health* (pp. 281-302). Orlando, FL: Academic Press.

Wortman, C. B., & Lehman, D. (1985). Reactions to victims of life crisis: Support attempts that fail. In I. G. Sarason & B. R. Sarason (Eds.), *Social support: Theory, research and applications* (pp. 463-489). Dordrecht, The Netherlands: Martinus Nijhoff.

Wright, P. (1979). Some recent developments in the sociology of knowledge and their relevance to the sociology of medicine. *Ethics in Science and Medicine, 6,* 93-104.

Wright, P., & Treacher, A. (1982). *The problem of medical knowledge: Examining the social construction of medicine.* Scotland: Edinburgh University Press.

Wuest, J. (1990). Trying it on for size: Mutual support in role transition for pregnant teens and student nurses. *Health Care for Women International, 11,* 383-392.

Yarcheski, A., & Mahon, N. (1989). A causal model of positive health practices: The relationship between approach and replication. *Nursing Research, 38*(2), 88-93.

Yoak, M., & Chesler, C. (1985). Alternative professional roles in health care delivery: Leadership patterns in self-help groups. *Journal of Applied Behavioral Science, 21,* 427-444.

Young, C. E., Giles, D., & Plantz, M. (1982). Natural networks: Help giving and help seeking in two rural communities. *American Journal of Community Psychology, 19*(4), 457-468.

Zachariah, R. (1985). Intergenerational attachment and psychological well-being during pregnancy. In R. A. O'Brien (Ed.), *Social support and health: New directions for theory and research* (pp. 168-174). Rochester, NY: University of Rochester Press.

Zarem, D. (1982). *Professional involvement with self-help groups.* Unpublished doctoral dissertation, University of California, Los Angeles.

Zimmerman, R. S., & Connor, C. (1989). Health promotion in context: The effects of significant others on health behavior change. *Health Education Quarterly, 16*(1), 57-75.

Index

About the Author

Miriam J. Stewart, B.Sc.N., M.N., Ph.D., is Professor in the School of Nursing and is cross-appointed as Professor, Department of Community Health and Epidemiology, at Dalhousie University, Halifax, Nova Scotia, Canada. She is the recipient of a scholar award from the Medical Research Council of Canada and the National Health Research Development Program for her research program. This program focuses on social support, self-care and coping, and salient interventions for diverse community and clinical populations: hemophiliacs with AIDS, the elderly with strokes, children with chronic illness, and family caregivers. The ideal relationship between self-help groups and health professionals also is under investigation. Her research has been presented at numerous national and international conferences. She is the primary author and editor of the book titled *Community Health Nursing in Canada,* published in 1985 by Gage Publications. She has published 40 articles and chapters dealing predominantly with social support, health promotion, primary health care, and social isolation. She is a frequent reviewer for peer-reviewed journals and for national funding agencies.